MR. FLEMING'S

HOW TO GROW AND USE GOURMET & MEDICINAL MUSHROOMS

A Mushroom Field Guide with Step-by-Step Instructions and Images for Mushroom Identification, Cultivation, Usage and Recipes

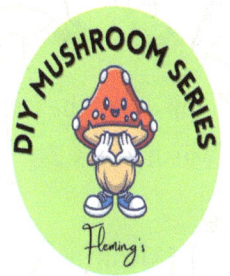

STEPHEN FLEMING

Chapters

Part 1

1. Welcome to Mushroom 101
2. Understanding The Science of Growing Mushrooms
3. Growing Mushrooms at Home
4. Mushroom Cultivation Techniques
5. What and How to Grow?
6. Dealing With Common Problems
7. Earning Profits by Growing Mushrooms
8. Frequently Asked Questions
9. Conclusion
10. Glossary

Part 2

1. Story of Healing Mushrooms- Otzi the Iceman to Alexander Fleming
2. Let's Meet 18 Medicinal Mushrooms
3. How Mushrooms Heal
4. Identifying/Foraging Top 7 Medicinal Mushrooms
5. How to Take Medicinal Mushrooms
6. How to cook Medicinal Mushrooms: 7 Recipes
7. Frequently Asked Questions (FAQ) & Glossary
8. Conclusion
9. Reference

PART 1

THE MUSHROOM CULTIVATION GUIDE

A Beginner's Bible with Step-by-Step Instructions to Grow Any Magical Mushroom at Home

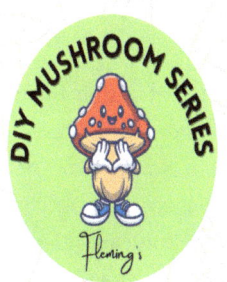

Stephen Fleming

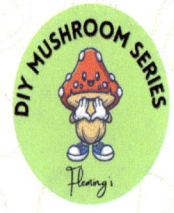

© Copyright 2021 - All rights reserved.

The content contained within this book may not be reproduced, duplicated or transmitted without direct written permission from the author or the publisher.

Under no circumstances will any blame or legal responsibility be held against the publisher, or author, for any damages, reparation, or monetary loss due to the information contained within this book, either directly or indirectly.

Legal Notice:
This book is copyright protected. It is only for personal use. You cannot amend, distribute, sell, use, quote, or paraphrase any part, or the content within this book, without the author or publisher's consent.

Disclaimer Notice:
Please note the information contained within this document is for educational and entertainment purposes only. All effort has been executed to present accurate, up-to-date, reliable, complete information. No warranties of any kind are declared or implied. Readers acknowledge that the author is not engaged in the rendering of legal, financial, medical or professional advice. The content within this book has been derived from various sources. Please consult a licensed professional before attempting any techniques outlined in this book.

By reading this document, the reader agrees that under no circumstances is the author responsible for any losses, direct or indirect, that are incurred as a result of the use of the information contained within this document, including, but not limited to, errors, omissions, or inaccuracies.

Words of Caution

- The contents of this book are for educational purposes and are not intended to offer personal medical advice.

- You should seek the advice of your physician or another qualified health provider regarding a medical condition. Never disregard professional medical advice or delay seeking it because of something you have read in this book. The book does not recommend or endorse any products.

- Any book, video, or other means of learning can't replace learning physically from an expert. These forms of information are only additional guidance to be used along with a practical demonstration and training.

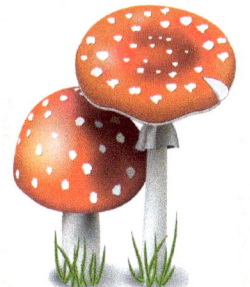

"from spore to spore, from dust to dust - in this whole world, mycelium we trust!"

Chapters

1. Welcome to Mushroom 101
2. Understanding The Science of Growing Mushrooms
3. Growing Mushrooms at Home
4. Mushroom Cultivation Techniques
5. What and How to Grow?
6. Dealing With Common Problems
7. Earning Profits by Growing Mushrooms
8. Frequently Asked Questions
9. Conclusion
10. Glossary

1. Welcome to Mushroom 101

Introduction

Humans have been consuming mushrooms for ages. Mushrooms come in a variety of shapes, sizes, and colors; depending on the species, they also vary in appearance. Some varieties are used in traditional medicine by various cultures across the globe. They are also commonly used as meat and seafood substitutes in vegetarian and vegan cooking. Mushrooms are rich in nutrients and antioxidants, are highly flavorful, and are an excellent source of *umami*, the fifth flavor (core fifth tastes including sweet, sour, bitter, and salty).

They can also be used medicinally for creating tinctures and teas. Mushrooms are the perfect low-cal and high fiber replacement for meats and seafood. Regular consumption of mushrooms is associated with better cardiovascular and brain health, weight loss, better skin, and even protects your body from certain types of cancer.

Mushrooms are primarily available in the wild and can be cultivated on farms, but mushrooms can also be grown at home, just like any edible plant or herb. What more? Growing mushrooms at home are cost-effective and make for a wonderful hobby.

For beginners, the first step is to understand multiple mushroom cultivation techniques thoroughly. There are different types of mushroom cultivation techniques such as making a grain spawn, PF Tek, five-gallon method, log grow, etc. Each of these techniques comes with its own set of benefits. In addition, depending on the method, the spawn and substrates used to grow mushrooms also vary.

In this book, you will learn in detail about all of this. Apart from this, you will also be introduced to the basics of mushrooms, their biology and life cycle, and how you can start growing some popular variants at home.

Once you understand this process, you can grow any mushrooms you aspire. By avoiding the common mistakes discussed in this book, your chances of success as a beginner also increase.

Once you get into the groove of mushroom cultivation, you can use it to create an additional stream of income as well.

The business side of selling mushrooms is also discussed in the later chapters. This book has different business ideas, from selling to local chefs and restaurants to set up your stall at the farmer's market.

As mentioned, mushrooms are a powerhouse of essential nutrients and vitamins. Apart from this, they are filled with beneficial active compounds with scientifically proven medicinal and healing properties.

Adding mushrooms to your daily diet is a great way to improve your overall health and wellbeing. From weight loss and better cardiovascular health to improved immune functioning and better cognition, the benefits of medicinal mushrooms cannot be overlooked. Once you get the hang of growing mushrooms at home, you can use that information for growing medicinal and psilocybin mushrooms.

This book will act as your guide to learn how you can grow delicious and exotic mushrooms right at home, just like people across the world have been doing for centuries. So, are you eager to get started and jump into the world of mushroom cultivation? If yes, there's no time like the present to get going.

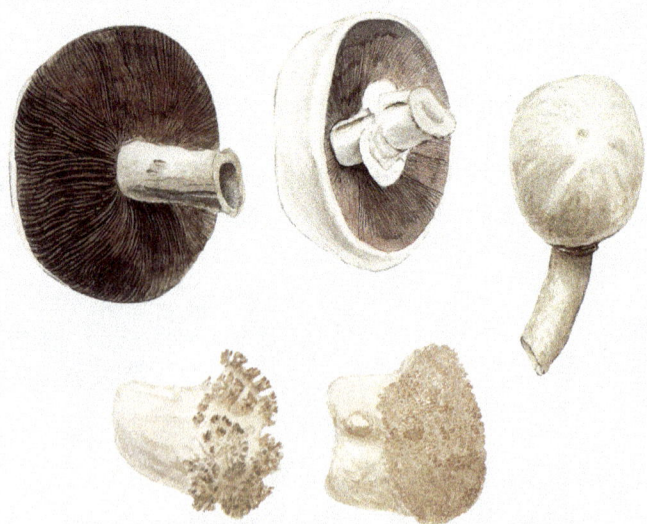

Vintage Photo - Edible Mushroom Types

Mushroom 101

What's the first thing that comes into your mind when you think of mushrooms?

You probably think about button mushrooms(champignon), enoki, or shiitake. Well, there's so much more to mushrooms than these three varieties. Most of us are familiar with mushrooms, but very few realize the diverse, helpful, and interesting benefits and uses they offer. The fruiting body that is visible and sprouts from a wide interconnected network of underlying root-like structures is known as a mushroom. Mushrooms come in a variety of sizes, shapes, and colors. Even their anatomy differs. Some types of mushrooms are edible, some have medicinal properties, and some are considered psychoactive while others are purely used for decorative purposes. Some mushrooms are incredibly toxic and poisonous as well. So, before you start growing mushrooms, it is important to understand a little about them.

They can also be used medicinally for creating tinctures and teas. Mushrooms are the perfect low-cal and high fiber replacement for meats and seafood. Regular consumption of mushrooms is associated with better cardiovascular and brain health, weight loss, better skin, and even protects your body from certain types of cancer.

Mushrooms are primarily available in the wild and can be cultivated on farms, but mushrooms can also be grown at home, just like any edible plant or herb. What more? Growing mushrooms at home are cost-effective and make for a wonderful hobby.

For beginners, the first step is to understand multiple mushroom cultivation techniques thoroughly. There are different types of mushroom cultivation techniques such as making a grain spawn, PF Tek, five-gallon method, log grow, etc. Each of these techniques comes with its own set of benefits. In addition, depending on the method, the spawn and substrates used to grow mushrooms also vary.

In this book, you will learn in detail about all of this. Apart from this, you will also be introduced to the basics of mushrooms, their biology and life cycle, and how you can start growing some popular variants at home.

Once you understand this process, you can grow any mushrooms you aspire. By avoiding the common mistakes discussed in this book, your chances of success as a beginner also increase.

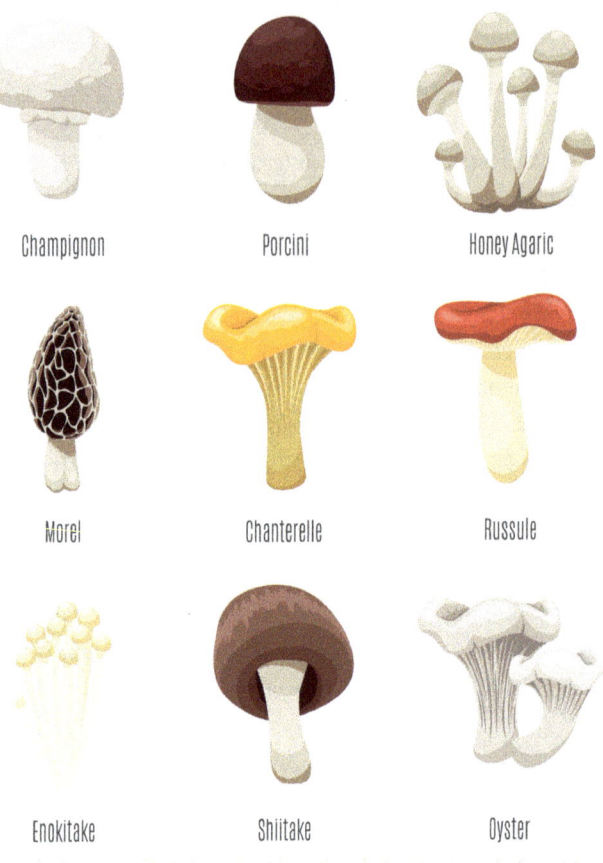

Majorly Cultivated Mushroom Types

Basics of Mushrooms

The reproductive structure produced by a specific type of fungi is known as a mushroom. It's quite similar to the fruit produced by plants. Instead of seeds, mushrooms have millions of microscopic spores present in the gills under the caps. These spores are spread by natural agents such as wind and animals that scatter them from one area to another. Once these spores land on a suitable substrate or food source, they germinate and form an intricate network of interconnected microscopic rooting threads known as mycelium, which penetrates their food source. The mushroom pops up and is visible above ground while the mycelium stays underground and persists for years together, extracting the nutrients available.

There are over ten thousand types of mushrooms that are currently known to us, and scientists believe this is just a fraction of what's present out there. General estimates range between 50,000-100,000 species that are yet to be identified. Yes, you read that right. Some of these varieties are excellent sources of nutrients or have medicinal properties, while others are highly toxic and even psychoactive.

Here is a fun fact – the largest living organism in the world is believed to be a fungus and is known as armillaria ostoyae. It is also nicknamed the humongous fungus. It covers almost four square miles and is larger than the largest mammal on this planet that is the blue whale. The Malheur National Forest in Oregon is its home. This fungus feeds on the roots of other trees in the forest and leeches all nutrients from them. It kills the trees by decaying them. This is the primary reason why the fungus has managed to grow to such humongous proportions. The part of the fungus that's visible above ground makes up only a small part of it, and most of its weight that is believed to be about 35,000 tons, is in the form of an underground mycelial network.

Mushrooms play different roles in the natural world. Some types of fungi promote the process of decomposition by devouring rotting wood, grass, and other organic matter. Some help trees extract nutrients and water from the soil while obtaining sugars and other carbohydrates they need to grow from the said trees.

Mushrooms can be helpful, they can form symbiotic relationships, and they can be parasitic as well. Some types of mushrooms attack tree roots or insects and devour them. Some mushrooms have medicinal applications as well. Apart from these helpful properties and nutritional profiles, there are different uses for them as well. Since most species of mushrooms are not yet known to us, every discovery is changing the perception of these fungi.

Some recent discoveries have helped scientists believe mushrooms can be used to clean landfills. The pestalotiopsis microspora is a species of mushroom that is fully capable of devouring or breaking down, and digesting polyurethane. Simply put, they believe this mushroom thrives by devouring plastic, which will certainly be a handy trait in today's world! When it comes to the wonderful world of mushrooms, remember that we have barely scratched the surface, and there is plenty to be discovered.

Foraging Mushrooms in the Wild

You can purchase mushrooms from a local grocery store or farmer's market. Another option is to grow them at home.

Apart from these two options, there is a third option you might not have thought of. This is to forage mushrooms in the wild. Certain types of mushrooms are rather tricky to grow at home and can only be foraged in the wild. Some popular edible mushroom varieties such as truffles, porcini, chanterelles, morels, and hedgehog mushrooms are quite difficult to grow at home.

That said, foraging mushrooms in the wild is not an activity that is recommended for the average Joe. You need to have a thorough knowledge of mushrooms, should be able to identify them without any doubt, and should know what to look for.

Certain mushrooms, especially the toxic ones, look quite similar to their edible counterparts. If you're not familiar with mushrooms or don't understand the natural habitat, growing conditions, and their appearances, chances are you will end up eating the wrong ones. This can prove fatal in most cases.

Another common problem you will encounter while collecting mushrooms in the wild is the scope of potential contaminants. They are a food source for different living beings including insects, critters, animals, and even other types of fungi. If you're not careful, you might end up biting into a wild mushroom that looks quite fresh on the outside, but when you look closely, it's riddled with worms and creepy crawlies on the inside. This might not kill you, but it will definitely kill your appetite.

These days, the world we live in is extremely polluted. Pollution is no longer restricted to cities and has seeped into the rural environment too. So, if mushrooms are growing in any or near polluted environment, they will absorb the toxins they're exposed to. Unfortunately, these toxins will find their way into your system if you're not careful.

You should also consider the seasons during which mushrooms grow in the wild. During certain seasons, you will come across plenty of mushrooms. But these mushrooms might not appear in the parts you discovered previously. Or even if they do, they might be infested. When you start cultivating mushrooms at home, you can avoid all of these issues. You also have a greater degree of control over environmental factors making it easier to grow higher yields.

Why Grow Mushrooms at Home?

If you are into gardening, growing mushrooms is a wonderful idea. Cultivating mushrooms at home is an incredibly exciting, fun, and satisfying process. As a beginner, prepare yourself to run into a couple of problems initially. As with any other skill, it takes plenty of effort, consistency, and practice to master the art of cultivating mushrooms at home. Once you get the hang of it, you can also cultivate them to earn profits.

Regardless of all this, remember it is a learning process. All your efforts will come to fruition when you can finally harvest the first flush of brilliant mushrooms. Whether it is a batch of shiitake or enoki, plucking mushrooms you grew is rewarding. This will also give you the motivation to keep going despite the potential obstacles you face.

An incredible advantage of growing mushrooms at home that cannot be overlooked is the variety it gives. When you walk into a grocery store, you'll have to choose from the mushrooms available in their produce section. When you start growing at home, you can pretty much yield whatever you want once you get the hang of it. From edible variants to medicinal ones, the choices are endless. Another advantage of growing mushrooms at home is it is cost-efficient. If you usually consume plenty of mushrooms, it can be quite costly, especially when you add the costs in the long run. The costs are even higher if you are looking for some rare varieties that aren't usually available in regular grocery stores and cost a pretty penny. You can avoid this by growing them at home. The initial costs are a little high but once you are investing in the required equipment and tools, you can keep growing multiple flushes.

Once you master the art of cultivating mushrooms at home, it can also become a source of income. If you are looking to create a supplementary or additional source of income, this will come in handy. Most of the edible varieties, especially the rare ones, are in high demand at farmer's markets and restaurants. If you get really good at growing them, you can sell them to local chefs or even start selling them at the farmer's market. You might not necessarily become rich but it is a great side hustle. This, coupled with all the information given in this book about setting up a mushroom business will certainly increase your earning capacity.

Apart from all these benefits, cultivating mushrooms is an incredibly interesting and satisfying process. Watching the mushrooms grow from their inoculation stage to seeing the mycelium colonize and the pins form to harvesting them, the journey is rewarding. It is not something that will happen overnight but your efforts will be worth the while. As with any other form of gardening, cultivating mushrooms is rewarding.

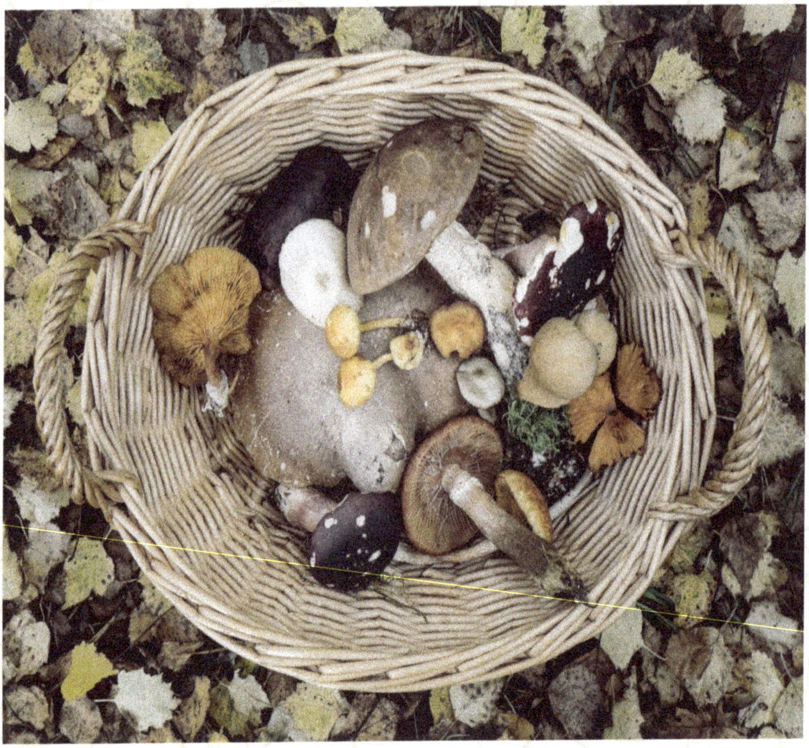

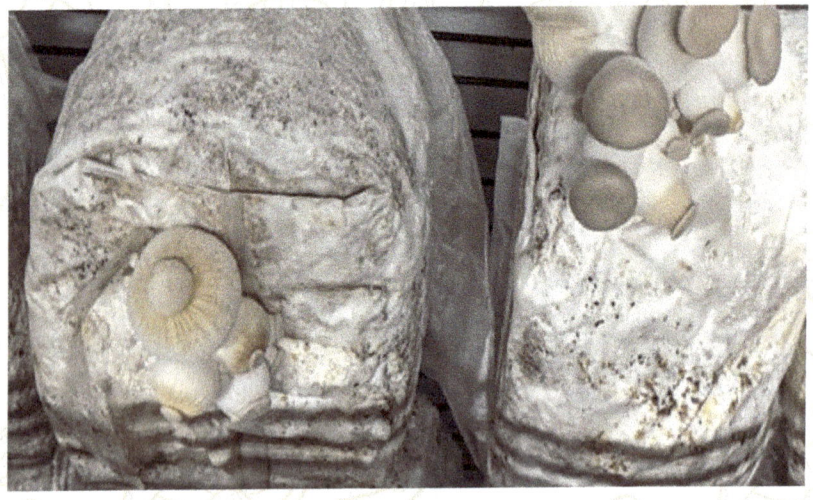

Foraging Mushrooms in Wild
(Photo by Andrew Ridley on Unsplash)

Growing Mushrooms at Home

Uses & Benefits of Mushrooms

Mushrooms are quite tasty and are commonly used as meat substitutes. They also have healing properties. Different types of mushrooms have been used in traditional medicine by various cultures across the globe. Whenever you are starting something new, looking at the benefits offered automatically increases the motivation to stick with the process. This stands true for cultivating mushrooms as well.

Here are some uses and benefits of mushrooms.

- **Reduces the Risk of Cancer**

The antioxidants present in mushrooms are believed to reduce the risk of breast, lung, prostate, and other types of cancer. This is believed due to the high level of selenium in them. Apart from this, mushrooms also contain Vitamin D. According to a study conducted by M. Rita I. Young and Ying Xiong (2018), Vitamin D supplementation can reduce and even treat certain types of cancer. Mushrooms also contain a helpful antioxidant known as choline. The findings of Shanwen Sun et al. (2016) suggest the consumption of choline and betaine can reduce the risk of cancer. The research was undertaken by Erin L Richman et al. (2012) supports the claim that consumption of choline reduces the risk of prostate cancer.

- **Better Heart Health**

Cardiovascular health improves when your body gets sufficient dietary fiber, vitamin C, and potassium. These healthy ingredients are present in mushrooms! Potassium helps regulate blood pressure and reduces the risk of hypertension. Sufficient consumption of vitamin C is also needed for maintaining heart health. The findings of Melissa A. Moser and Ock K. Chun (2016) show a direct risk between lower levels of vitamin C intake and cardiovascular diseases. The research conducted by Petr Sima et al. (2018) shows that the consumption of a specific type of fiber known as beta-glucans reduces the levels of cholesterol. Well, you don't have to look any further because most edible mushrooms contain plenty of beta-glucans.

Mushrooms promote better heart health because they can be used as a replacement for salt. Instead of using table salt, start using mushrooms as a substitute. Their natural umami and savory flavor will instantly enhance the taste of any dish you are cooking without harmful sodium. An entire cup of mushrooms hardly has around 5 mg of sodium. The glutamate ribonucleotides present in mushrooms make them a healthy replacement for salt.

- **Reduces the Risk of Diabetes**

Type-2 diabetes is a rapidly growing global health concern. This condition is characterized by elevated levels of blood sugar, which is beyond your body's ability to manage. Type-2 diabetes is a risk factor for several cardiovascular disorders too. Consumption of dietary fiber is believed to reduce the risk of diabetes by regulating blood sugar levels. The research conducted by Marc P. McRae (2018) shows that the consumption of dietary fiber reduces the risk of type-2 diabetes. Mushrooms, as you must already know, are a great source of dietary fiber.

- **Slows Aging**

The most common cause of aging is oxidative damage caused by free radicals in the body. A straightforward solution to reverse this process is reducing oxidative damage. This function is performed by antioxidants. Mushrooms are rich in two specific antioxidants known as glutathione and ergothioneine. The findings of Michael D. Kalaras et al. (2017) support the common notion that mushrooms are extremely nutritious and contain helpful antioxidants. When your body gets a sufficient dose of these antioxidants, the visible signs of aging, such as wrinkles, are reduced. So, if you want healthy, glowing, and supple skin, increase your intake of mushrooms.

- **Better Brain Health**

The helpful antioxidants present in mushrooms tackle inflammation. Inflammation and oxidative stress are the common causes associated with cognitive decline. The simplest way to reverse this is by increasing your intake of antioxidants. Mushrooms are rich in antioxidants, and their regular consumption will improve your brain health. According to the study conducted by Michael D. Kalaras et al. (2017), antioxidants, especially ergothioneine and glutathione, present in mushrooms improve cognitive functioning and brain health. A study conducted by Lei Feng et al. (2019) suggests the consumption of mushrooms improves cognitive functioning while reducing the odds of cognitive decline.

- **Stronger Bones**

Vitamin D and calcium are two essential nutrients needed for maintaining and strengthening your bones. Mushrooms are an incredible source of both these essential nutrients.

They contain a compound known as ergosterol that is converted into vitamin D during maturation when exposed to sufficient light. The consumption of mushrooms gives your body its daily dose of vitamin D and calcium.

- **More Energy**

Mushrooms are rich in a variety of B complex vitamins such as B1 (thiamine), B2 (riboflavin), B3 (niacin), B5 (pantothenic acid), and B9 (folate). B-complex vitamins play a crucial role in your body – the production of red blood cells. These cells are responsible for transporting oxygen to different cells in the body. They also promote better conversion and utilization of the energy from the food consumed. Mushrooms also contain vitamin D, minerals such as selenium, potassium, copper, iron, phosphorus, calcium, zinc, magnesium, and choline. When your body gets its daily dose of nutrients, then its functioning improves too. A combination of all these factors will automatically make you feel more energetic.

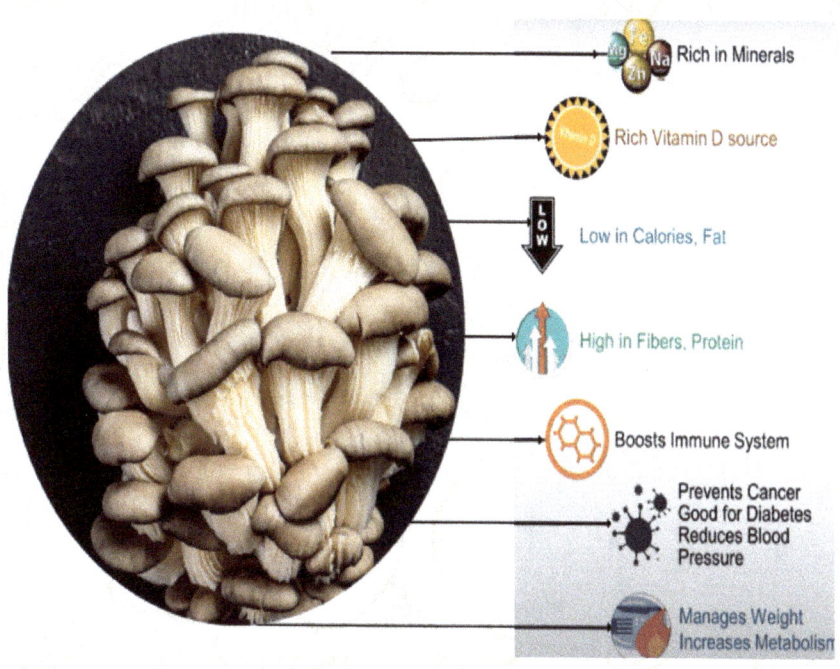

Benefits of Mushroom

2. The Science of Growing Mushrooms

Before you start growing mushrooms, learning about their basic components, types, and life cycle is important. This gives you better insight into the type of mushrooms you are growing and how to grow and take care of them. Understanding the basic biology at play goes a long way while cultivating mushrooms at home.

Start With the Anatomy of Mushrooms

There are different types of mushrooms, and their anatomy varies depending on the variety. Having said that, most mushrooms have the same parts as the ones discussed in this section.

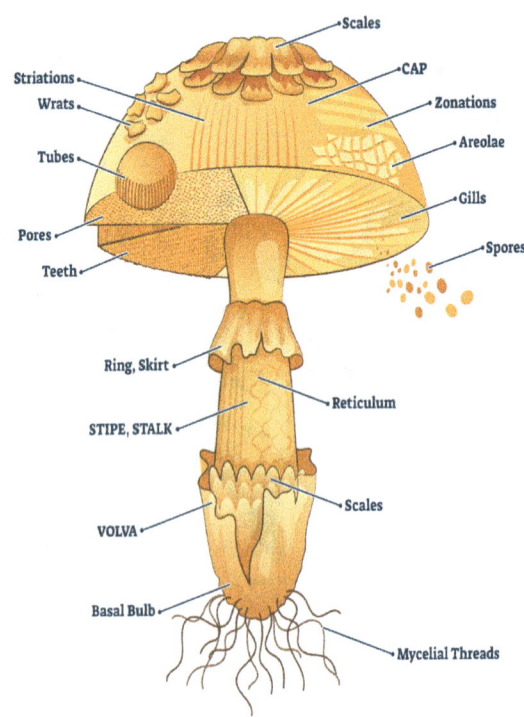

Cap

The cap or the pileus refers to the top part of the mushroom. This is the first thing you will notice whenever you look at a mushroom. As the name implies, it refers to the dome or umbrella-like structure and is the outer part of the mushroom. Umbrellas shield us from the rain and harsh sun. Similarly, the mushroom's cap also protects the spores and gills from harsh elements.

Spores

Spores or pores are found in the gills. Flowering and fruiting plants usually produce seeds for propagation, whereas mushrooms produce spores. They are the mushroom's means of reproduction.

Mycelium

Plants have roots that burrow into the earth to obtain the nutrients they need. Similarly, even mushrooms have fine hair-like strands growing downward into the soil to obtain the nutrients they need. The mycelium in mushrooms functions just like the roots of a plant. They also help new mushrooms grow under favorable circumstances. This makes up for most of the structure of the fungus growing underground or any other substrate that acts as their food source.

Fruiting Body

The entire mushroom sprouting from the mycelium is known as its fruiting body. It usually contains gills, stipe, veil, volva, and cap.

Stipe

The stipe is also known as the stem. This refers to the vertical portion of the mushroom on which the cap rests. The stem is visible above the surface. In the wild, wind acts as a vector that helps scatter the spores for propagation. For this, the cap and gills must be above the surface and high enough, so the spores don't drop to the ground and are instead carried away.

Ring

The annulus of the mushroom is commonly known as the ring. It is a small part of the veil left on the mushroom stem. Think of it as an additional layer of protection for spores that keep growing when mushrooms are still developing. As the cap starts growing, it breaks through the veil. The leftover of this process forms the ring around the stipe.

Veil

A protective layer on the underside of the mushroom cap is known as the veil. This is where the spores are stored until they reach maturity. The cap starts flattening out as the mushrooms grow and mature. Once this happens, the veil breaks so the spores can be released.

Volva

Most mushrooms have a cup-like structure close to their base known as the volva. This is the remainder of the veil enclosing the spores.

Hyphae

The mycelium is made of fine filament-like structures known as hyphae.

Types of Fungi

As we know currently, there are more than ten thousand different types of mushrooms around the world. It might seem like a significant number, but mycologists believe it's only a fraction of the types of mushrooms left to explore. All these mushrooms can be divided into four broad categories or species known as saprotrophic, mycorrhizal, endophytic, and parasitic. This classification is based on how the mushroom obtains its sustenance or, simply put, how it feeds itself. Learning about these classifications will also make it easier while foraging mushrooms in the wild.

Saprotrophic Mushrooms

These mushrooms feed on decaying or decomposing matter known as detritus. So, they are referred to as natural decomposers. The digestive enzymes and acids produced by saprotrophic fungi help digest dead tissue including nonliving organic matter into smaller absorbable molecules of energy. So, plants, wood, animals, and any other type of organic matter become sustenance for these mushrooms. Mold and bacteria, the most common contaminants, also belong to the family of saprotrophs.

Saprotrophs play an important part in the food chain. Are you wondering how this is possible? Well, think of all the dead matter on the ground. If there were no organisms that recycle and decompose it, the forest floor would soon be covered with waste. Since saprotrophs derive their sustenance from decaying and dead tissue, they help clear the ground. They are extremely effective when it comes to breaking down complex organic matter and recycling it into nutrients that go back into the ecosystem. They are not only an important part of the carbon cycle through nutrient conversion but are an equally important part of the food chain as well. Saprotrophs include a variety of gourmet and medicinal mushrooms.

The most common saprotrophic mushrooms are morels, reishi, white button, shiitake, maitake, turkey tail, shaggy mane, black trumpet, giant puffball, oyster mushroom, chicken of the woods, and the yellow houseplant mushroom.

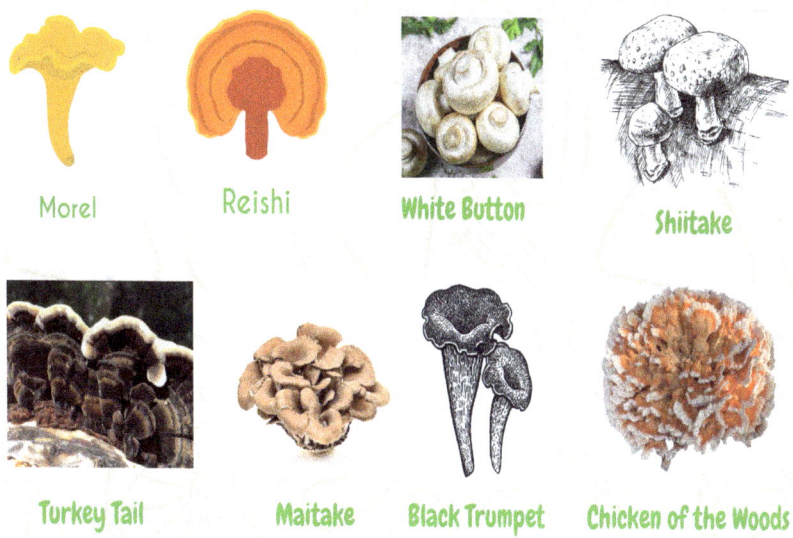

Morel   Reishi   White Button   Shiitake

Turkey Tail   Maitake   Black Trumpet   Chicken of the Woods

Mycorrhizal Mushrooms

Most mushrooms share a fascinating relationship with their surrounding or neighboring flora. This class of mushrooms has a symbiotic relationship with plants and trees. Mycorrhizal fungi play an essential role in soil composition and chemistry, including their nutrient profile. The mycelia of Mycorrhizal fungi create a symbiotic relationship with plants by weaving their way into root cells or wrapping themselves around the roots. This provides the plants with additional nutrients and moisture needed for their growth. In addition, the fungi obtain sugars such as glucose produced by the host. This not only helps the plants grow but sustains the development of the fungi as well.

The mushrooms produced by these fungi aren't easy to cultivate and are found only in the wild. However, the most common mushrooms belonging to this category are also the most delicious ones, including porcini, truffles, Caesar's mushrooms, matsutake, and chanterelles.

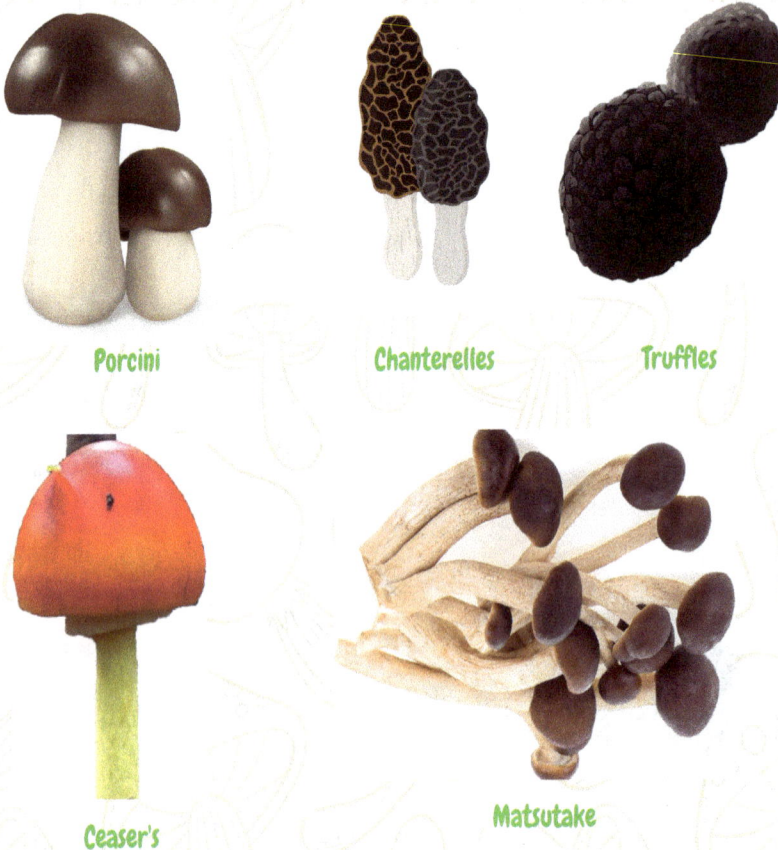

Porcini Chanterelles Truffles

Ceaser's Matsutake

Parasitic Mushrooms

There is a relationship between most mushrooms and the plants they grow on. That said, not all relationships are beneficial. As the name suggests, parasitic fungi obtain their sustenance by feeding on their host. In some cases, it also means a slow death for the host. The most common host for mushrooms are plants. Parasitic mushrooms usually enter the plant through any opening present in the leaves, lenticel, or even stoma. Parasitic fungi also have an interesting relationship with insects. Some can enter the insect and feed on it without killing it such as the Cordyceps militaris. The fungus enters its host and stays there until it is ready to release spores. The dried remains of the insect and this type of mushroom are used in traditional Chinese medicine.

The most common parasitic mushrooms are caterpillar fungus, Chaga, honey fungus, and lion's mane.

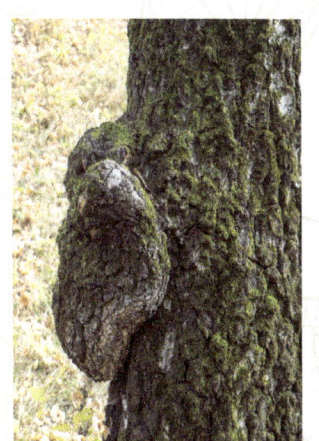
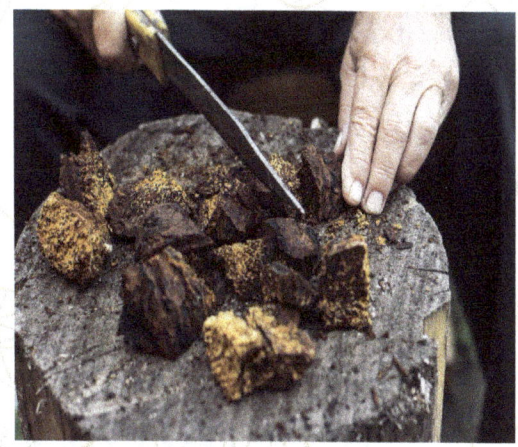

Chaga Mushroom

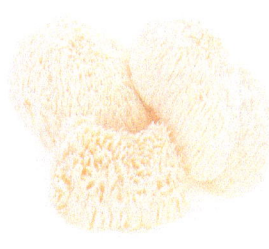
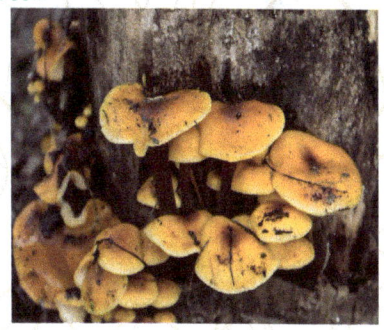

Lion's Mane

Honey Fungus

Endophytic Mushrooms

Some mushrooms don't belong to the categories mentioned above and exhibit unique characteristics that they deserve their separate category. These types of mushrooms create a partnership with plants, just like parasitic mushrooms. Unlike the latter, the former doesn't invade the tissue of its host. The host, in this case, not only remains healthy but benefits from the mushrooms too. The nutrient absorption and the host's resistance to pathogens increase with these types of mushrooms.

There isn't much known about the specific category of mushrooms. Most fungi in this category don't produce mushrooms, and their relationship with the host or plants is not yet understood fully. A common belief among mycologists is that specific types of saprophytic and parasitic fungi can reveal themselves to be endophytic with further research.

Mushroom Life Cycle

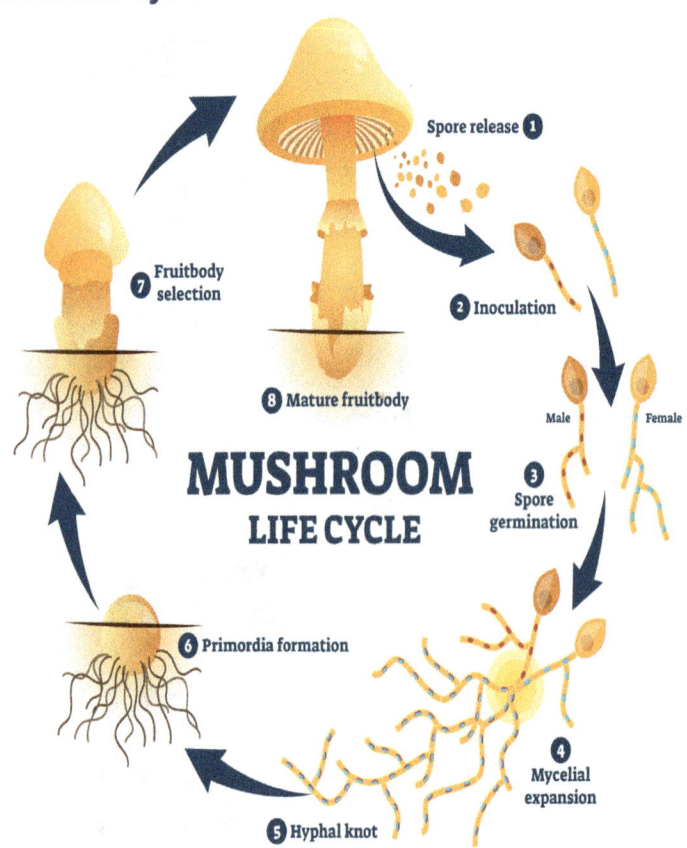

Before you learn to grow mushrooms, familiarizing yourself with their life cycle and basic reproduction is needed. This information gives you a better idea of what you can expect as the mushroom starts growing. For instance, some varieties of mushrooms can grow within a day while others take longer. The environmental requirements also differ from one mushroom to another. Most mushrooms require a steady source of moisture.

The life of a mushroom starts when the spore germinates. This happens only when the spore finds a suitable source of nourishment known as the substrate. The substrate varies from one mushroom to another. For example, a living insect or a tree would be a substrate for parasitic mushrooms, while soil or wood for others. As this spore germinates, the mycelium starts growing through the substrate. The digestive enzymes released by the mycelium help break down the nutrients available and transform them into absorbable energy for growth.

The mycelium keeps growing until the existing conditions are suitable for fruiting. The mushroom or the visible fruiting body is the sex organ of the mycelium. It contains spores that contain the required genetic material for reproduction. Mushrooms reproduce sexually and asexually. If the hyphae of two genetically unique mycelia of mushrooms of the same species are combined, they fuse into a single adult mycelium. This is known as the sexual reproduction of the mushroom.

The spores are the gametes in mushrooms. They are present within the pileus and are located right under the mushroom cap. The underside of the cap in most mushrooms is lined with fine tooth-like structures known as gills. The gills radiate symmetrically from the stipe and are lined with basidia. The basidia for each of the gills contain four spores each. Each of these spores, in turn, is composed of a single cell that can easily sustain harsh conditions.

Here is a fun fact about mushrooms!
A single mushroom is capable of producing 31000 ballistospores every second. This means a single mushroom can produce up to 2.7 billion spores daily. The genetic material present within each spore is slightly different from the other. This variation makes the progeny slightly different from the parent fungi. When mushrooms start growing, this variation can be easily regulated and minimized through cloning. While cloning, only the desirable traits of the selected mushrooms are propagated.

The spores of the mushroom don't automatically start growing once they are released. Instead, they live dormant until they find the right substrate to obtain the required nutrition and wait for suitable climatic conditions.

Once they have reached this stage, the entire process starts again. The spores germinate and produce mycelium. Hyphal knots are produced whenever the mycelium is ready to fruit. Hyphal knots are also known as primordial and are commonly referred to as pin sets or pins. The primordial starts dividing and branching at a cellular level and grows into different parts of the mushroom resulting in its familiar structure of cap, gills, stem, and so on.

The total number of cells present in the primordial is the same as the ones in a mature mushroom. These cells start absorbing water and, therefore, expand in size. Mushrooms are made up of up to 90% of water and this is one of the reasons why mushrooms seem to appear rather quickly after a rainfall. As a mushroom starts expanding, its cap that is usually rounded, to begin with, starts flattening. The rounded cap contains the spores and gills that the whale protects. As the cap flattens, the veil pulls away from the stem and eventually breaks away from it. This allows the spores to be released.

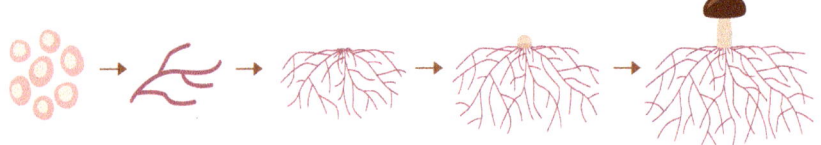

Mushroom Life Cycle

3. Growing Mushrooms at Home

Now that you are aware of how mushrooms grow, let's get to the exciting part – growing mushrooms at home. There are two different options available when it comes to growing mushrooms at home. You will also need different items and equipment to grow them properly. The steps followed for growing mushrooms vary from one type to another. That said, some basic steps are commonly used for growing most types of mushrooms.

So, are you eager to start growing mushrooms at home?

DIY vs. Growing Kits

The two standard options available when you want to grow mushrooms are to start by purchasing a kit and using it or gathering the required supplies and doing it yourself.

There are pros and cons to each of these methods. What you are hoping to get out of the entire experience will determine the best way for you. Here are the pros and cons of using a grow kit and the do-it-yourself (DIY) approach.

Using a Grow Kit

There are several varieties of grow kits easily available these days. You can use them for cultivating just about any mushroom you want at home. The grow kits come with ready-to-use colonized or inoculated substrates. Once you have the kit in place, you need to introduce the spawn at the right time and maintain the ideal fruiting conditions. Once all these things are in place, they will start fruiting.

One of the most important advantages of using a grow kit is it's incredibly easy to use and a lot cheaper than doing it yourself. If you want to go with the DIY option, be prepared to invest your time and money into this process. Because you will need to make the substrate, sterilize it, wait to inoculate it, create a fruiting chamber, and not to forget, purchase all the required equipment.

That said, this advantage is also a drawback. Whenever you want to grow, you will need to purchase another kit and start all over again. Once you are aware of the process and have gathered the supplies, it becomes easier to grow mushrooms again and again.

Apart from it, the yield of mushrooms produced by a grow kit cannot be compared with the ones produced with a reliable mushroom DIY growing technique at home. If you are just getting started with it or want to experience the process of growing mushrooms, using a kit will be quite easy.

Choosing a grow kit will give you a rough idea of the overall cultivation process. If you are interested in simply trying the process or seeing if you like it, purchase a kit and get started.

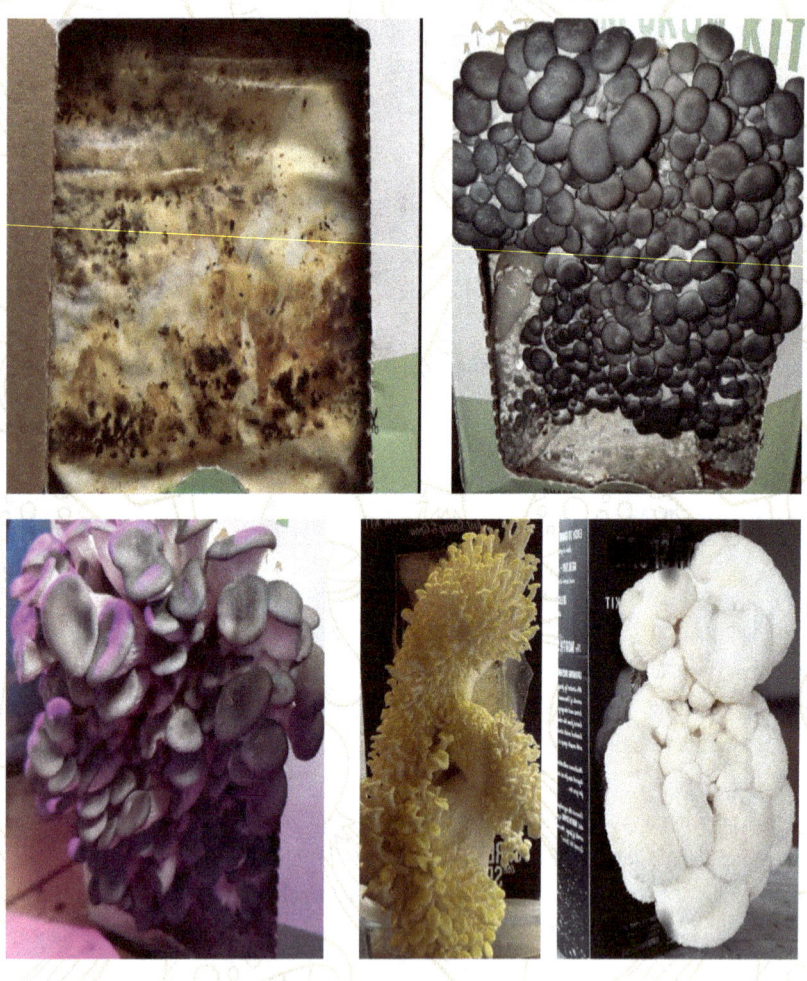

Variety of Mushroom Growing Kits

Doing it Yourself

If you are interested in learning something new and want to familiarize yourself with cultivating mushrooms at home, doing it, yourself is the best option available. This is also a good option if you like building things on your own and want a hands-on approach. After all, when you have to start from scratch, the knowledge and experience you gain are invaluable. This can be used for the subsequent growth of mushrooms as well.

The primary concern you must be aware of while opting for the DIY route is the time and effort it involves. The initial startup costs and the time commitment cannot be ignored. You will need to select a substrate, prepare the substrate, ensure everything is sterile, and create the ideal fruiting chamber.

Even if you are thinking of learning mushroom cultivation as a hobby, considerable time and effort are needed. Apart from it, there is also the risk that you will not get it right in the first go. Even if you have prepared the substrate properly, not sterilizing it can quickly derail the process. Growing mushrooms is a process of trial and error. If you are invested in it and don't mind the effort, opt for the DIY option.

Other considerations that can derail the process include preparing a poor substrate or accidentally contaminating the substrate. You can either view this as a drawback or a learning experience. If you think of it as a learning experience, the entire process becomes engaging and rewarding.

Now, let's consider the benefits of the DIY approach. A significant benefit of choosing this approach is the yield it offers. You can consistently grow one large yield after another once you know how to go about it. This by itself is incredibly rewarding. Another advantage is that you are learning something new. This skill can be transformed into a hobby. If you become good at it, you can also turn this hobby into an additional stream of income. You will learn about creating an additional source of income from mushroom cultivation later in this book.

When compared to the cost of purchasing a kit, the DIY approach is costlier. This is because you need some basic equipment. Even though the startup costs are high, you can use them for growing multiple batches in the future. For instance, the fruiting chamber, mason jars, and the pressure cooker used don't have to be discarded.

Instead, you can use them for future grows too. Once you have the required supplies on hand, you simply need to purchase other single-use items such as the required substrate, rubbing alcohol, and gloves. You will try growing the limited set of mushrooms available by using a grow kit. However, if you are interested in producing higher yields and mushrooms that are more delicious than those available in a kit, do it yourself.

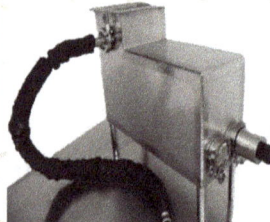
DIY Steam Generator

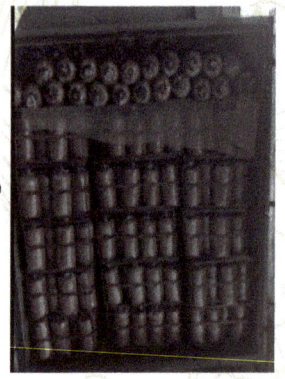
DIY Bulk Pasteurization

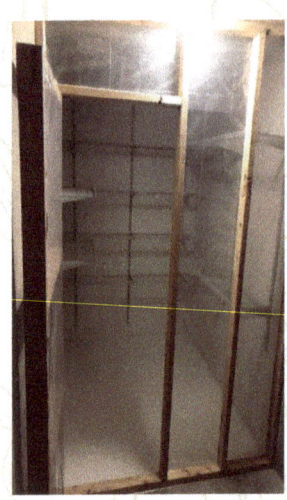
DIY Growing Chamber

Growing Mushrooms on Your Own

You will need some basic supplies if you want to start growing mushrooms at home. The supplies depend on the process you want to follow, along with the mushrooms you want to grow. So, the items you will need to purchase or gather will vary. That said, here are some basic items you will need.

Equipment and Items

Spores

Mushrooms grow from spores, and therefore, you will need spores or a culture. The spores can be obtained in the form of a spore print or a syringe. Using a spore syringe is a better idea because it is easy to handle, but inoculation also becomes easier.

On the other hand, using a spore print gives you more growth than a syringe. Depending on the effort you are willing to make, you can either opt for a syringe or a print.

You can also purchase a readymade mushroom culture or colonized substrate if you want to reduce the time involved in the cultivation process. Mushroom mycelium that is suspended on an agar plate or in a liquid is known as a culture. Spores take a while to germinate. You can easily bypass this waiting period by using culture for inoculating multiple substrates.

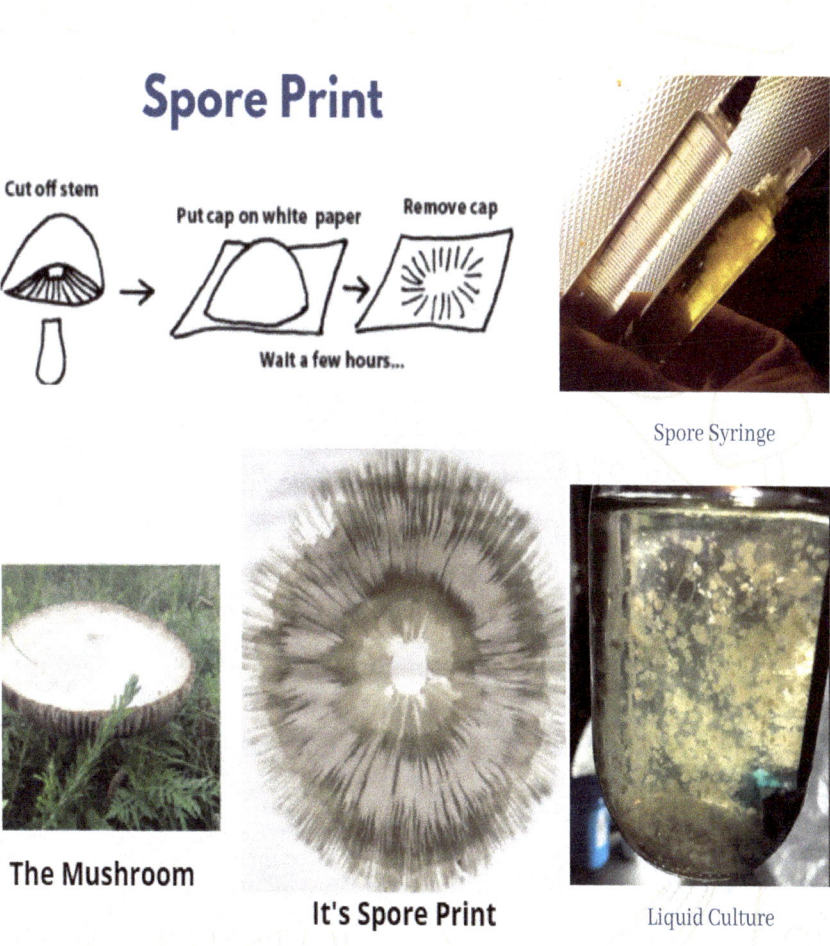

The Mushroom | It's Spore Print | Liquid Culture

Syringe

You will need a syringe to inoculate the substrate unless you decide to use agar. Usually, in mycology, a 10-CC syringe with a 1.5-inch 16-gauge needle is recommended. Readymade syringes can be reused easily. However, don't forget to sterilize them between uses. You can use a pressure cooker to sterilize them or fill them with boiled water. So, it is important to purchase syringes that are heat resistant

Agar

Agar is used to isolate the mycelium before inoculation. This step is optional. That said, a little extra effort goes a long way when it comes to cultivating mushrooms. With this bit of action, the result will be much better. You will learn more about using agar for cultivation later in this book.

One of the Agar Recipes :

- 1100 ml Water
- 21 grams Agar
- 11 grams Dextrose
- 4 grams malt Extract
- 4 grams Yeast Extract
- 6 grams Peptone

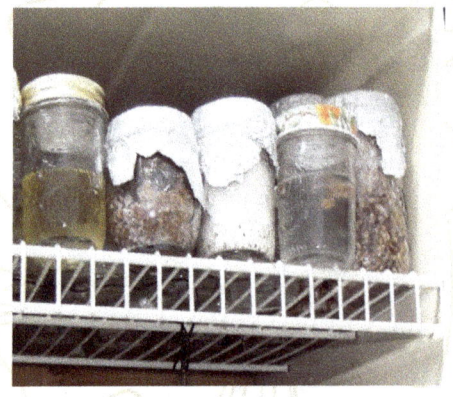

Petri Dishes having Spawn, Liquid Culture and Agar ,

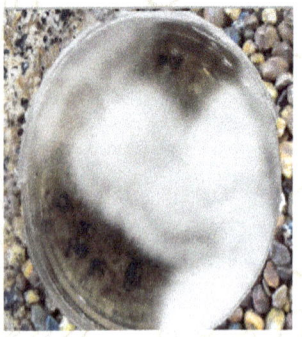

Agar Culture

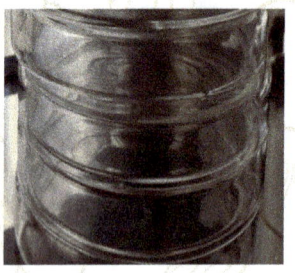

Glass Petri Dishes

Petri Dishes

You will need Petri dishes to prepare the culture. Alternatively, cups, mason jars, or any other flat container of your choice can be used too. Remember that the container you choose should be such that it can be covered and sterilized. As long as the container meets both these requirements, it's all good.

Pressure Cooker

Sterile technique is essential when it comes to growing mushrooms. You will learn about this later in this chapter. Different methods can be used for sterilizing the substrate that doesn't include a pressure cooker. You can also use a pot for boiling and steaming the required equipment. That said, a pressure cooker is the best option because it ensures any bacterial or yeast contaminants present are thoroughly destroyed. If there are any contaminants, it will ruin the growth.

Mason Jars

A heat-resistant container with a lid is needed for sterilizing and pasteurizing substrates. Mason jars are the perfect fit for this process, but the receptacle used will depend on the growing method you follow. That said, for most grows, you will need jars of one type or another.

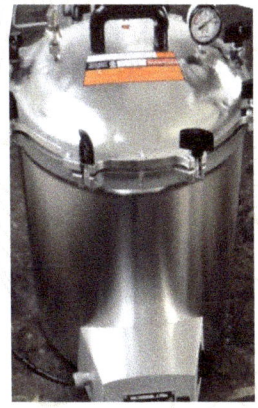
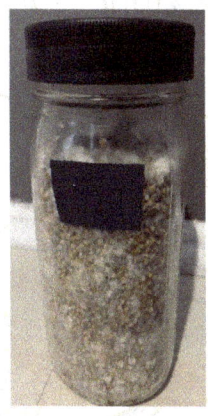
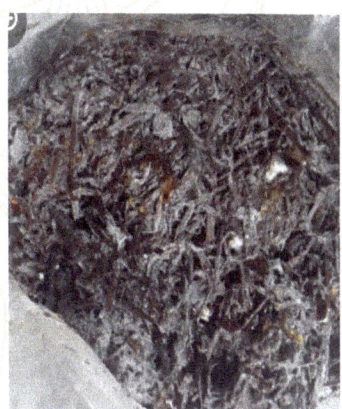

Pressure Cooker   Mason Jar   Substrate

Growth Substrate

Depending on the mushrooms you want to grow, the growth substrate will also vary. In addition, the preferred food source for mushrooms differs according to their type. Wood, grains, compost, seeds, and dung are the most commonly used substrates to grow mushrooms.

Perlite

Mushrooms need a humid environment to thrive, and perlite creates the perfect growing conditions.

The perlite needs to be soaked in some water. After this, use it to line the bottom of the fruiting chamber. This helps create an ideal humid environment for the mycelium.

After this, the mycelium starts fruiting. Once again, all of this will depend on the type of mushroom you're growing and where you are growing. For instance, if you are growing mushrooms outdoors, you don't need perlite.

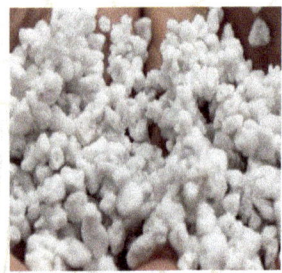 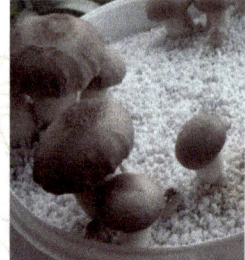 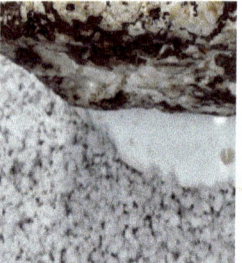

Perlite

Glove Box

The importance of keeping all the equipment used sterile cannot be overstated. By using a glove box, you can ensure the entire process is sterile. On average, up to 10,000 fungal spores are present per cubic meter of air. These fungal spores and other environmental contaminants can derail the growing process. To avoid this, you need a glove box. Not using a glove box increases the risk of growing undesirable mold instead of the mushrooms you had in mind. You can either purchase the glove box or make one at home with basic materials.

Here is a simple glove box you can make at home using basic materials.

First, you will need a clear storage bin with a lid. It should be big enough to hold at least 60 quarts, a pair of gloves, epoxy or any other strong glue, and a tube of sealant. You will also need a measuring tape, a sharp knife/blade or a rotary tool, and a marker.

Now, let's get started. Start by gathering the required supplies. The clear plastic storage bin should be see-through. Don't opt for an opaque box because you will not see what's happening on the inside. You can easily purchase this at a local supermarket, hardware store or even order it online.

Use the measuring tape and mark a point about 4-inches from the left and right sides of the container. Using the felt pen, mark a 4-inch diameter circle on either side of the box. The size of the holes should be such that your arm fits through it. Use the compass or the rotary tool to outline the circle.

Use the razor knife or any other sharp blade to cut holes using the outline traced in the previous step. You can stop at this step and your glove box is ready. Always wear gloves while handling the substrate in this box. To make it even better, insert the gloves you decide to wear into the holes you have cut. The gloves should be placed such that about 2-inches of them still stay outside the box. This material outside the box can be glued to the side using strong glue. After the glue dries, go around the outer and inner sides of the gloves using a layer of sealant or silicone. This creates an airtight chamber in the container to reduce the risk of contamination. Simply place your hands through the gloves to handle the substrate. The gloves chosen for this process should be loose-fitting such as large kitchen gloves.

Here is a simple glove box you can make at home using basic materials.

First, you will need a clear storage bin with a lid. It should be big enough to hold at least 60 quarts, a pair of gloves, epoxy or any other strong glue, and a tube of sealant. You will also need a measuring tape, a sharp knife/blade or a rotary tool, and a marker.

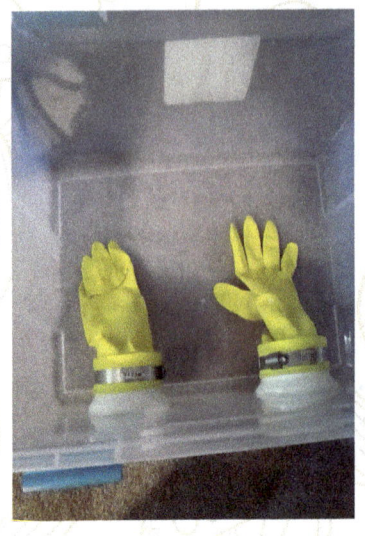 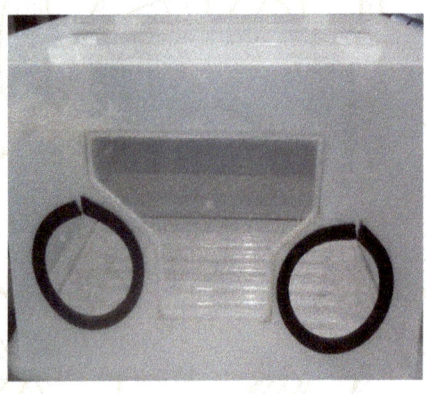

Glove Box

Gloves

Even if you are using a glove box, it is always better to use disposable gloves while handling everything inside it. This ensures you have created a sterile environment free of all contaminants. You don't necessarily need to wear sterile gloves. Just ensure that you thoroughly rub down the gloves with 70% isopropyl alcohol or hand sanitizer before working with them.

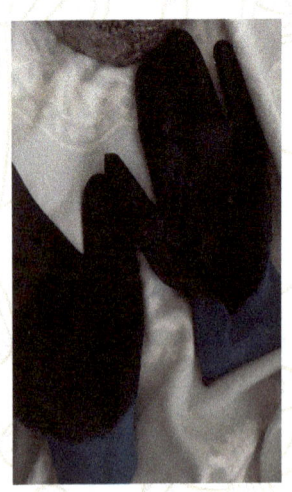

Gloves

Rubbing Alcohol

You need to be incredibly careful while growing mushrooms. A little carelessness means you have left the doors wide open for different contaminants to take a hold of the mushrooms you are trying to grow. Whenever you are making a mushroom spore print, inoculating, or are in general handling anything associated with growing mushrooms, keep the surfaces as sterile as possible. So, you need to clean the glove box using Lysol or 10% bleach solution. You should do this before introducing the culture or substrate for inoculation as well. Apart from it, don't forget to sanitize your gloved hands and any other tools used in the process.

Lighter

If you are using a syringe to inoculate the jars, you will need a lighter or a Bunsen burner. Use the lighter or the burner to heat the tip of the syringe until it is glowing hot. Whenever you need to inoculate between different jars or even inoculate at different points, repeat this step to reduce the risk of contamination.

Fruiting Chamber

Some methods of growing mushrooms don't need a fruiting chamber. Most of the popular strains of mushrooms, especially if you want to grow them indoors, need a fruiting chamber. You will learn more about making a fruiting chamber at home in the subsequent sections.

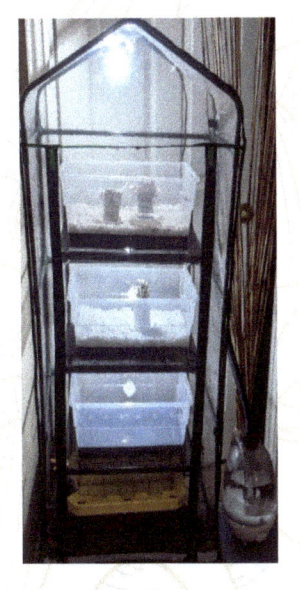

Air Box Fruiting Chamber

Martha Chamber

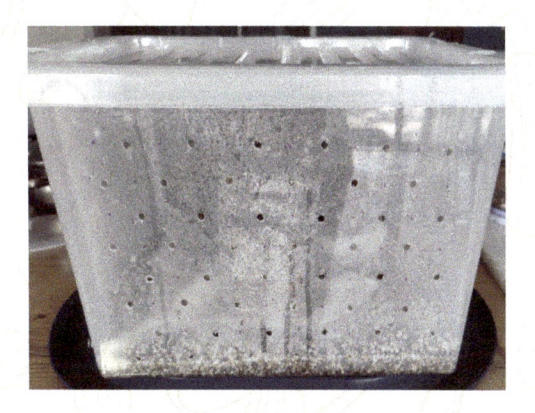

Steps to Follow

Several growing techniques can be used according to the type of mushrooms you want to grow. From using jars to growing mushrooms on outdoor patches and fruiting them on logs, multiple options are available. Laying down the exact process, you'll need to follow is not possible without determining the type of mushrooms you want to grow, the substrates you want to use, and the technique you wish to follow. That said, here is a general outline of the basic steps you will need to follow.

- **Start by Selecting a Mushroom Type**

The substrate you wish to use to the environment needed for mushrooms starts with the type of mushroom you want to grow. Unless you know the type or variety of mushrooms you are trying to grow, you cannot move on to the other steps. Read about the basic methods that can be used to produce the mushrooms and pick a variety that suits your type. There are different things to consider, from understanding the best or ideal growing location and the substrate you want to use to the difficulty of cultivating the mushrooms. Well, you don't have to spend more time looking for the different types of mushrooms you can grow at home because they will be discussed in the next chapters.

- **Select a Substrate**

As mentioned, the substrate will vary depending on the mushrooms you want to grow. Some mushrooms prefer grains, while others need wood. Straw, vermiculture, and dung, or a combination of all these, can also be used as a substrate. Depending on the type of the mushroom, we will also come across different types of substrates that can be used along with the techniques involved.

- **Preparing the Substrate**

Once you have chosen a substrate, it must be prepared so you can start cultivating mushrooms. The method of preparation also varies according to the type of substrate you have chosen. Usually, to prepare the substrate, place it in a mason jar with the required water. After this, the jars need to be pressure cooked at 15 PSI (pound-force per square inch) to ensure they become sterile. This also depends on the substrate you are using. For instance, if you are growing mushrooms on a log, this step isn't needed.

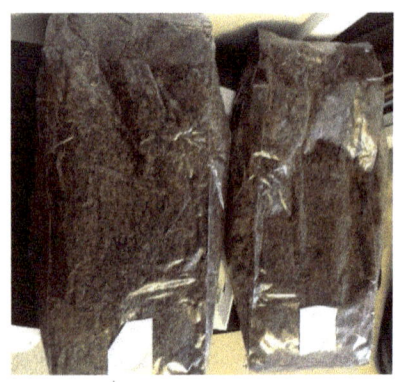

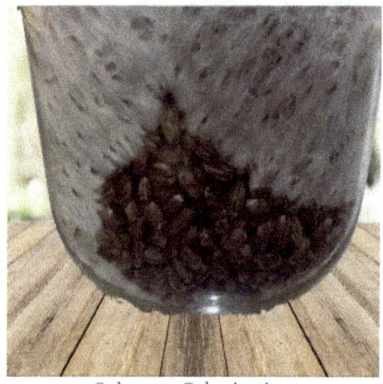

Substrate   Substrate Colonization

The Inoculation Starts

If you were using mason jars for inoculation, then place the jars into the glove box. First, ensure the glove box is thoroughly cleaned. To this, you can either use a solution of bleach or Lysol. After this, inject the spores directly into the substrate. Alternatively, a colonized piece of agar can also be placed in it. Once again, this varies depending on the technique you want to use.

Substrate Colonization

The duration of the colonization process depends on the culture along with the type of mushroom you want to grow. Depending on whether you are using a liquid culture agar or spores, the time taken for incubation varies. This period is crucial for the growth of the mushroom. The environmental conditions, especially the temperature and moisture level, must be closely monitored for the substrate to colonize.

Birthing the Spawn

A fully colonized substrate is known as the spawn. You can either mix this spawn with the growing medium of your choice, such as coir, or directly shift to the fruiting stage. Once again, this depends on the growing technique you are following. The spawn must be placed in the required fruiting environment to start fruiting.

Mushroom Pinning

The mushroom pins start developing depending on the type of mushroom you are growing and the technique used. From a few weeks to a couple of months, mushrooms can take their own sweet time. So, this step is all about patience. This is also an exciting phase in the growing process. Once the pins start developing, they will be ready for harvest within no time.

Harvesting the Mushrooms

Once the mushrooms you are growing have matured, it is time to harvest them. This is when all your efforts come to fruition. Harvesting the fruits is quite easy and incredibly rewarding. Simply pinch the mushroom at its base, twist it slowly, and pull them. This is how you harvest most mushrooms

Whenever you are harvesting, try to gather as much of the visible portion of the mushroom without damaging its mycelium as possible. Once the mushrooms are harvested, you can consume them immediately or store them for later. To prolong its shelf life, you can dry or freeze them depending on the mushroom variety you have grown.

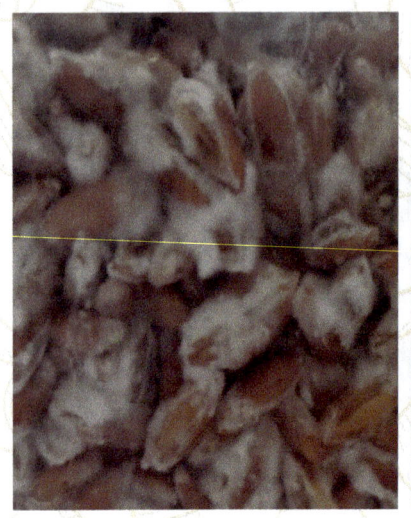

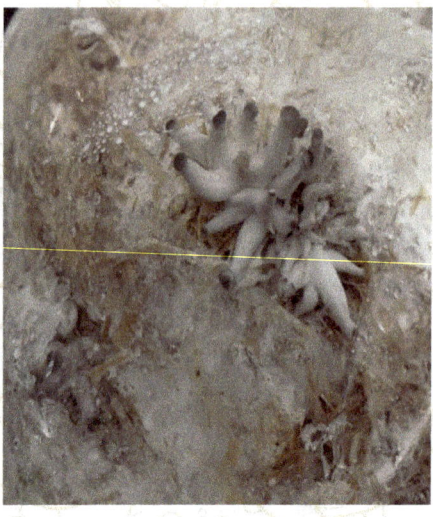

Birthing Spawn   Mushroom Pinning

Keep Things Sterile

The substrate is the most critical part of the cultivating process because this creates an environment the mycelium needs to grow. A primary problem you will need to deal with here is contamination due to bacteria, mold, or even other types of undesirable fungi. This happens because the substrate offers a moist and nutrient-dense environment for other contaminants as well. If any of these undesirable contaminants take hold of the substrate, you will need to start again. If these contaminants grow and spore, it will ruin the current batch and make future cultivation difficult.

This is one of the reasons why you need excellent sterile techniques while cultivating mushrooms at home. Depending on the type of substrate you are using and its density, the substrate must be pressure cooked at 15 PSI for 60- 90 minutes.

You should also ensure the instruments, tools, and equipment used in this process are thoroughly cleaned. Don't forget to sanitize your hands and always scrub the glove box before using it. Initially, it's always better to make a little extra when it comes to sterilization. When you keep cultivating mushrooms, you will better understand this process and can also develop a proper technique. As long as you properly sterilize the substrate and ensure everything is clean, you will have a nice and healthy spawn that will give you a good harvest.

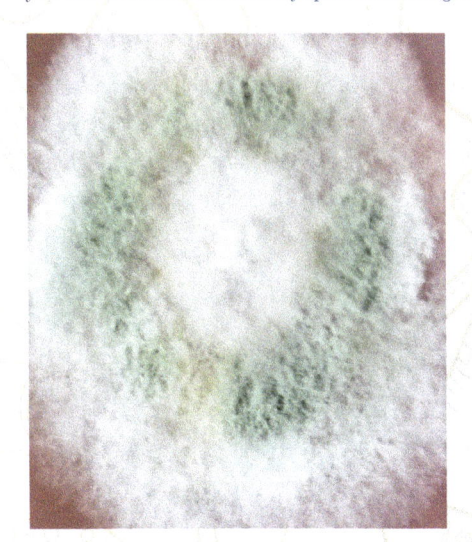

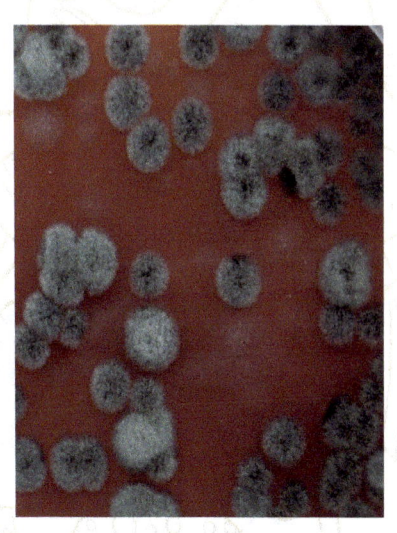

Contamination (Green Mold) in Substrate

Common Contaminants

While growing mushrooms, the common contaminants you need to watch out for are mold or fungal contaminants, bacterial contaminants, and pests. Here is how you can learn to identify each of these contaminants.

Mold or Fungal Contaminants

Mold or fungal contaminants are not only difficult to deal with, but they mean the entire batch is ruined. They present themselves as discoloration or even fuzzy white growth on the substrate or spawn. The most common fungal contaminants include cobweb, pink, green, black, blue-green, and dry bubbles.

Bacterial Contaminants

Bacterial contamination is characterized by yellow lesions or blotches toward the edges or on the caps. Bacteria are airborne and commonly occur during the fruiting stage. Therefore, if the fruiting area is too moist or humid, it increases the risk of bacterial contamination. To reduce this risk, ensure there is sufficient fresh air circulating through the area you have chosen and reduce the humidity levels.

Wet spot or sour rot is the most common type of bacterial contaminant. It not only looks bad but, as the name suggests, smells quite bad too. The batch is compromised if you notice any gray and slimy presence in the substrate, with a foul odor reminiscent of dirty socks. To avoid this, the substrate must be soaked for 24-hours before sterilization. This lets the dormant spores germinate, making it easier to kill them during sterilization.

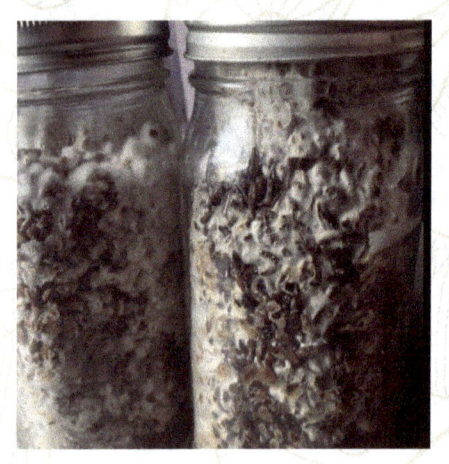

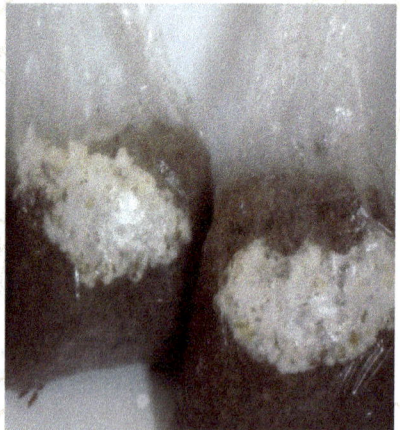

Bacterial Contamination

Pests

Different types of insects are known as pests, and they feast on the mycelium and the mushroom itself. Even though they might not necessarily ruin the harvest, they are a nuisance, to begin with. Mites and fungus gnats are the most common type of pests mushrooms are susceptible to. Mites feed on the mycelium and damage it.

They are also responsible for the discoloration of mycelium. By keeping the grow area thoroughly sanitized and clean, you can avoid them. Gnats are tiny flying insects that harm mushrooms. They start tunneling through the flesh of mushrooms and create open spots that leave them more prone to further contamination from other pathogens such as bacteria. Gnats are incredibly easy to identify because they look like fruit flies. To avoid these critters, practicing thorough sanitization is needed.

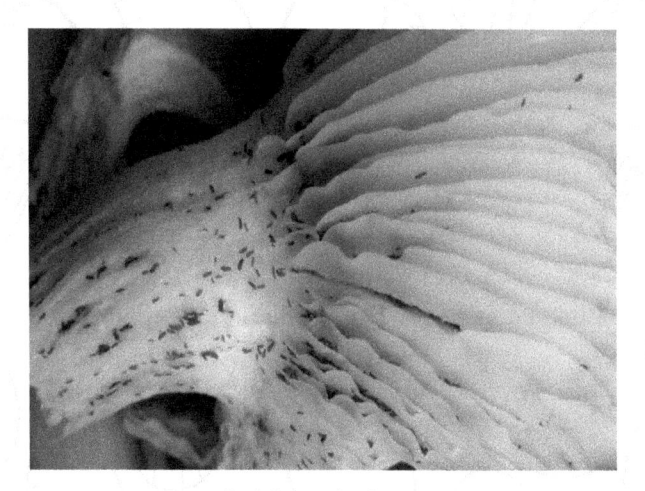

Pest Contamination

Mushroom Growing Environment

Before you go ahead and learn about the different cultivation techniques that can be used for growing mushrooms, it's important to determine where you want to grow them. Different factors have to be considered before you make this decision and let's learn about them.

- **General Climatic Conditions and Season**

Consider whether you live in a dry or humid environment. You should also consider the season for growing mushrooms. For instance, mushrooms thrive after rains. Similarly, when the weather is too hot and dry during the summer months, it is not the right time to grow mushrooms because mycelium can die. Consider the usual temperature in the area you live along with the rainfall it receives.

- **Space Available**

Now, it's essential to consider the space available for growing. For indoor cultivation, the relevant questions would be :

- Do you have sufficient space indoors to grow mushrooms?
- Can you create a fruiting chamber within your home?
- Do you have any additional closet space for growing mushrooms?
- Given your living situations, would it be ideal to grow outdoors or indoors?

If you want to grow outdoors, you need to consider a suitable and appropriate space for the mushrooms. For example, do you have a backyard? Or do you have a yard or an outdoor space for creating a mushroom patch?

- **Type of Mushrooms and Indoor/Outdoor Cultivation**

Now, you should start considering the different types of mushrooms you want to grow.

To do this, first, you have to decide the growing environment to be indoor or outdoor?

For both cases, you have to consider many important factors like :

- Conducive environment for fungi growth?
- What is the desired yield you are expecting?
- Are there any specific humidity and temperature requirements for the said mushrooms?

Factors for Indoor Cultivation

- What is the size of yield you want to grow?
- Is it possible for you to grow outdoors in a giant patch?
- Are you interested in mushrooming just to get the hang of it?
- Or are you interested in growing pounds and pounds of mushrooms?
- Do you have any storage facilities for the harvest?
- Do you want to sell your harvest, or is it for personal use?

Now let's get to the most critical consideration of all. It is time to determine the growing method you want to use.

For example, do you think you can use an indoor fruiting chamber, or would it be better to grow the mushrooms outdoors?

Spend some time and carefully consider all these factors. Once you have answered these questions and have thought about them, you'll have a reasonably good idea of whether grown indoors or outdoors would be suitable. Let us consider both the indoor and outdoor options.

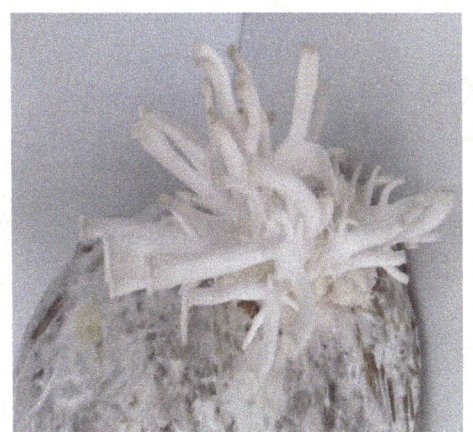

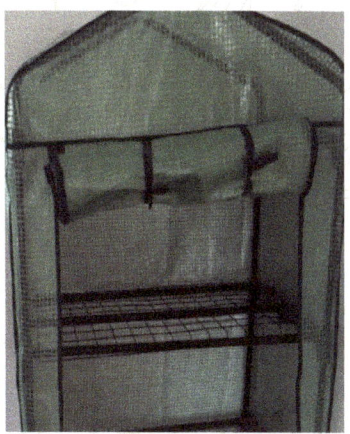

Indoor Cultivation

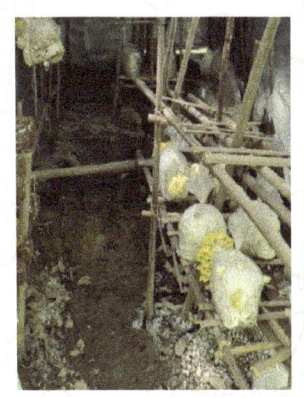

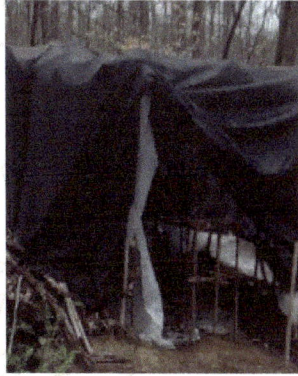

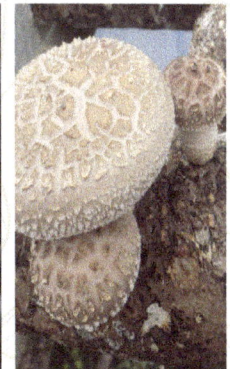

Outdoor Cultivation

Growing Outdoors

There are different reasons why cultivating mushrooms outdoors is a brilliant idea. For instance, certain species of mushrooms require plenty of air circulation. Therefore, they cannot grow in an environment with excess carbon dioxide buildup; that usually happens when you start growing indoors. If there is excess CO_2 or insufficient oxygen, the yield and the appearance of mushrooms will be affected. On the other hand, blue oyster and king oyster mushrooms thrive when grown outdoors.

The yield produced when you grow mushrooms outdoors is higher than the indoor options. Also, many varieties of mushrooms love oxygen, and all the extra oxygen they are exposed to outdoors gives you healthier and bigger mushrooms.

If you have a spacious yard outside, obviously, the yield produced there will be greater than any obtained from an indoor fruiting chamber. A large yard means you can create a large mushroom patch resulting in a large yield. This is ideal, especially if you want to start a mushrooming business.

That being said, deciding to grow mushrooms outside has a couple of disadvantages. The biggest factor is you cannot fully regulate the climatic and environmental factors outdoors.

Depending on the climatic conditions of the area you live in and the season you want to grow in, growing outdoors is not always an option. Unreasonable weather such as a cold spell or a heat wave can kill the mycelium in most species of mushrooms. Another factor you cannot ignore is humidity. If the area is quite dry, especially in a desert environment, growing outdoors is problematic. Finally, you cannot overlook the risk of pests while growing outdoors. Birds, common insects, worms, rabbits, and other creatures can feast on the fungi you are working hard to grow.

Apart from all these factors, it would help to consider the variety of mushrooms you want to grow. Unfortunately, it is not possible to grow all types of mushrooms outdoors. Some species thrive outdoors, while others require controlled humidity and temperature.

Here are the general steps you will follow while growing mushrooms outdoors.

The first step of getting started is to find the right location. Next, you will need a place for setting up the mushroom bed. To create a mushroom bed, you will need a raised bed-like structure. Ensure the mushrooms will not be exposed to too much sunlight and opt for a shady area or spot such as one under trees.

Once you have a spot, start by laying down wood chips and spawn. The most common type of wood chips you can use is the one used for smoking meat.

As long as the wood chips are not treated with any chemicals, they are ideal for growing mushrooms. First, lay down a single layer of wood chips along the cardboard lining of the bottom of the bed. Once the first layer of wood is laid, place the fully colonized mushroom spawn. You will learn more about making mushroom spawn in the following chapters under the heading, "Grain Spawn."

Once the spawn is in place, cover it with another layer of wood chips. you will need to keep repeating this process. It's quite similar to making lasagna. If the raised bed is about 13 square feet, you will need 6.5 lbs. of spawn. The top layer of the bed should be covered with wood chips and ensure the spawn is not exposed.

Once all these things are in place, it is time to cover the mushroom bed. The simplest way to cover the bed is by using a layer of straw. This prevents the bed from drying while keeping the elements away. It also acts as an additional layer of insulation. Once you have covered it with straw, soak the bed with water. You can use a water hose to do this. The moisture from the water will keep the bed moist for a couple of weeks at least but you will need to rewarm it to ensure the mycelium has sufficient moisture.

If you allow the bed to dry out, the mycelium cannot grow. You can also use shade cloth for additional protection and for creating the required shade for the mushrooms to grow.

Watering the bed once a week is a good idea if you live in a relatively dry area. On the other hand, keep an eye out on the bed if the site gets plenty of rain. If it looks like the bed is drying, water it. If it seems too moist, it can increase the risk of contamination. After a couple of months, if you look under the straw, you can see a layer of mycelium. It will take around six months until the pins appear.

The ideal time to harvest mushrooms is before they become too big. Once the caps are fully open, they become prone to contamination. Also, mushrooms start deteriorating rapidly once fully mature. Gently grip the mushroom along the base while gently twisting and pulling it. Harvest the mushroom when they are relatively young, after the first flush. The bed will produce a couple of more flushes until the substrate is fully spent.

If you want the bed to keep producing consecutive harvests, feeding it is essential; this means you will need to keep adding fresh layers of wood chips. However, you don't necessarily have to keep adding more spawns every year. The mycelium from one grow cycle will help reestablish another cycle of mushrooms. Add wood chips to the top of the bed and shuffle it with a rake to mix the chips with existing mycelium in the bed. After this, regularly water the bed for more mushrooms!

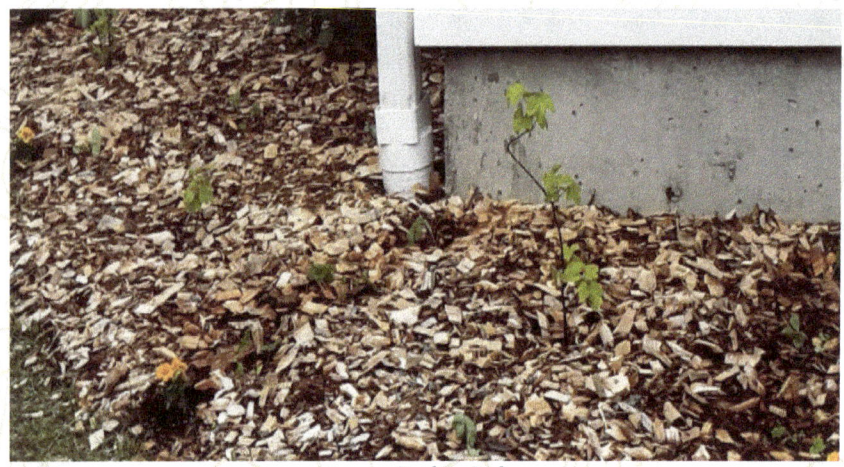

Outdoor Bed

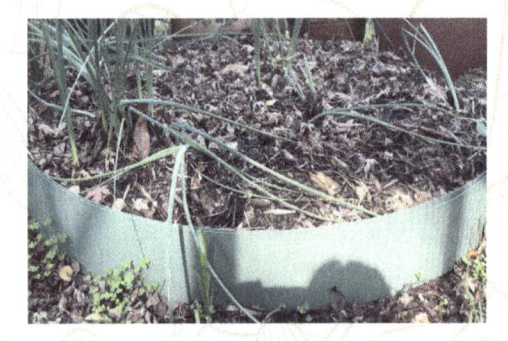

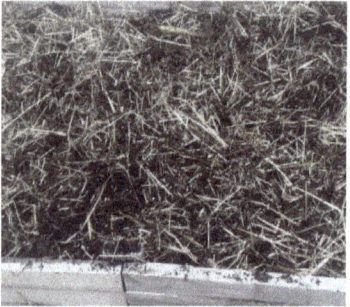

Raised Mushroom Bed

Growing Indoors

Forget about building a mushroom patch if you decide to grow indoors. The yield might be smaller when compared to the outdoor patches, but it gives you better control over the environmental factors. This means you have better chances of growing different types of mushrooms even if they have specific needs. You have complete control over crucial cultivation factors such as general humidity and temperature when you start growing indoors. Some mushrooms thrive in tropical and hot environments, while others require colder temperatures.

When you are growing mushrooms outdoors, the mushroom patch is subject to various environmental factors. These factors are redundant when you decide to grow them inside the house. While growing indoors, most species of mushrooms can be easily cultivated regardless of the season. Whether you want to grow mushrooms during the hot summers in Nevada or the cold winters, you can create the ideal temperature indoors.

Another important benefit of growing mushrooms indoors is it becomes easier to reduce the risk of contamination and avoid pests altogether. When mushrooms are grown outdoors, they become a tempting snack for different types of critters and pests. You will still have to deal with contaminants such as gnats, bacteria, and mold, but they are safe from critters and other creepy crawlies such as worms and insects.

If you decide to grow indoors, you need a specific area to grow mushrooms. In most cases, you will need a fruiting chamber. The good news is, making one at home is incredibly easy. Regardless of how big or small your home is, you can grow mushrooms without any hassles.

Even if it's a studio apartment, a fruiting chamber hardly takes any space and you can cultivate mushrooms within no time. Remember, the only condition is to select a spot or a place that doesn't get extremely cold or hot. For instance, if the attic becomes extremely hot during the days and the garage becomes cold at night, this is not the ideal spot for growing mushrooms.

Other factors you must consider growing indoors include air circulation and the light available. Mushrooms don't need much light to grow, unlike plants. That said, they need a little light because it determines the direction in which they grow. Light is also needed for pinning. If you are growing in a dark space, using a small compact fluorescent or a LED light will meet the lighting requirements. If you take a little extra precaution, you can start growing in small spaces even with poor ventilation. You need to ensure there isn't excess carbon dioxide buildup because it hurts the yield and increases the risk of contamination. Using a fan helps dispel excess co2 and provides the culture with the required air.

The ideal places to grow mushrooms indoors include the attic, garage, basement, cupboards, closets, or any other area that isn't regularly used. The selected space should be such that the fruiting chamber fits in it.

Fruiting Chamber

The term fruiting chamber has been mentioned repeatedly until now. If you are growing indoors, you need a fruiting chamber. Let's look at the different options available for building a DIY fruiting chamber within no time.

Shotgun fruiting chamber

A shotgun fruiting chamber is ideal if you want to use PF Tek and a couple of other growing techniques. You will learn in detail about the different techniques to cultivate mushrooms in the next chapter. For now, let's get back to building fruiting chambers.

Materials and Tools Needed

Here are the materials and tools you will need to build a shotgun fruiting chamber.
- One 60-quart clear plastic storage bin with a lid
- Kitchen strainer
- Perlite (10-12 quarts)
- Hygrometer (this is optional and is used to check the humidity levels in the fruiting chamber)
- A spray bottle
- Tape measure
- Power drill with a 1/4th inch drill bit
- Marker or a pen

Steps to Follow

The main component of a fruiting chamber is a clear plastic bucket or container with a lid. You can also use a clear storage bin. You can use any container that fits these requirements available at home or purchase one. The size of the container determines the size of the chamber, so it can be as big or small as needed. If you want, you can also use a mason jar as a fruiting chamber! According to this, the amount of perlite required will also vary. As long as it is a clear container with a lid, you can move on to the next step.

Now, it is time to start drilling holes into the container to promote air circulation. Take the tape measure and mark spots that are 2-inch apart in a grid-like manner.

Holes need to be drilled on all six sides of the container, including the top and bottom. Don't worry about the perlite falling through the bottom because wet perlite clumps together.

Once you have marked the spots, it is time to drill some holes. Fix the drill with a 1/4th inch drill bit and drill away. Ensure that you don't press too hard on the container while drilling holes because it can cause cracks. If any excess plastic is sticking out from the drilled spots, cut it away with a blade or a knife to create an even surface. Ensure that you have drilled holes in all the spots marked on all sides of the container.

Take a big enough strainer to hold the perlite you will be using in the fruiting chamber. Place the perlite in it, and put the strainer under running water. When you place the perlite under running water, it helps clean the perlite, infuse it with moisture, and remove any bits of dust that might have settled on it. Let the perlite soak in it and then drain the excess water. Don't leave it out for too long because it starts drying as well. To further sterilize the perlite, adding a little hydrogen peroxide to the water helps.

Once you have washed and cleaned the perlite, add it to the fruiting chamber. You need sufficient perlite such that it creates a 3- 4-inch layer at the bottom of the chamber. If you don't add sufficient perlite, it reduces the humidity in the chamber. If you are using a hygrometer, it will come in handy right here. Ensure the humidity level is between 80- 90% on the hygrometer.

This is the final step. Now that the fruiting chamber is ready and you have added the perlite to it, it's time to add the colonized cakes. Line the mycelium cakes with aluminum foil at the bottom to prevent contamination when they directly come in contact with the perlite. Ensure the perlite doesn't directly touch the exposed part of the mycelium cake. If this happens, it increases the moisture the culture is exposed to along with the risk of contamination.

You can spray water using the spray bottle if the chamber looks too dry. To determine whether sufficient humidity is present in the chamber, check whether water droplets have formed on the chambers' sides. Don't forget to fan the chamber to provide sufficient air circulation regularly. This also promotes fruiting. The fruiting chamber should be placed such that it doesn't get any direct sunlight. If you are using an artificial light source, opt for a fluorescent bulb. Ideally, the fruiting chamber should be exposed to 12 hours of sunlight or natural sunlight and should spend the rest time in darkness.

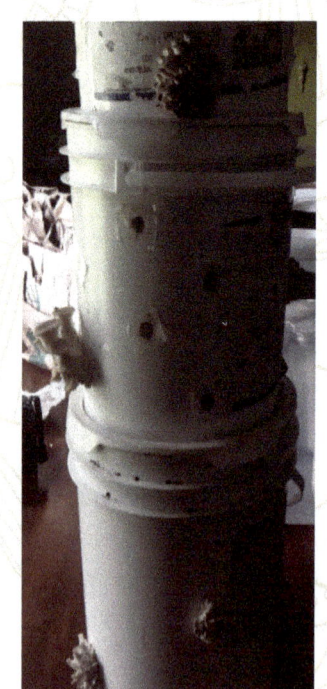

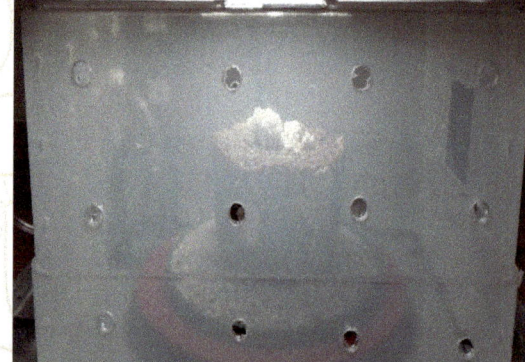

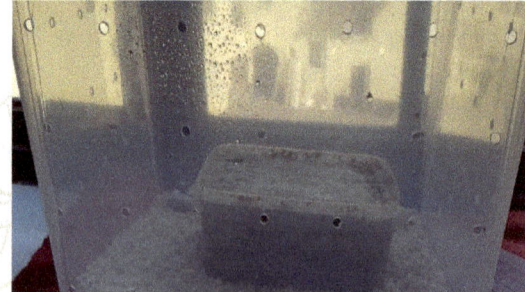

Shotgun Fruiting Chambers

Monotub

One of the most popular fruiting chambers commonly opted for by mushroom cultivators is a monotub. This is also incredibly easy to build at home. As with a shotgun fruiting chamber, even this has a large clear plastic storage bin. You will need to drill large holes along the four sides of the bin, excluding the top and the bottom. The bottom of the tub will be lined with the colonized substrate. The moist substrate provides the required humidity to grow mushrooms. When compared to a shotgun fruiting chamber, a monotub provides better results.

Materials and Tools Needed
Here are the materials and tools you will need

- A large clear storage plastic bin with a lead
- Micropore tape or polyfill
- Duct-tape (this is optional and helps secure the micropore tape or polyfill in place)
- Plastic-safe black spray paint (optional)
- Power drill or a sharp knife
- Marker or a felt-tip pen
- Tape measure

Steps to Follow

The size of the container will depend on the yield you want to obtain. Generally, it's better to purchase a storage bin with a lid that can hold at least 60 quarts. Remember, the container should fit in the space you want to grow. Don't opt for an opaque container and select one made of clear plastic.

Now, you need to line the bottom of the storage bin. This prevents any extra light from entering the bin. Light decides the direction in which the mushrooms grow. If you don't line the bottom of the bin, chances are the mushrooms will start growing toward the sides instead of the bottom. If they grow towards the side, it is known as side pinning. Along the bottom half of the tub, you can apply thick plastic tape to cover every square inch. Alternatively, you can also choose to spray paint the plastic container. Another option is to line the bottom of the container with a black plastic bag such as a trash bag. To make cleaning easier after the mycelium is spent in a growing cycle, use a trash bag to line the bottom of the bin.

Use the tape measure and marker to mark the spots for drilling holes. There aren't any strict rules about the placement of holes for air circulation in this method. The holes should be around 1.5-2-inches in diameter and spaced equidistantly. Drill three holes on the long sides and two on the shorter. The holes should be drilled vertically on the shorter side and horizontally along the longer sides.

Once you have marked the holes, it is time to drill or cut them. You can use a drill with a 2-inch saw-hole attachment. If not, you can use shears, a razor knife, or any other sharp blade to carve out the holes. Ensure that you are careful while handling the sharp blades because an accidental slip will leave you with a nasty cut.

Now, you have come to the final step of creating a monotub. You need to start covering the holes. There are two options you can use to cover the holes. You can opt for polyfill or micropore tape. While using polyfill, simply stuff the hole until it's tightly filled with the cotton-like material. If you are using micropore tape, you simply need to cover the holes using sufficient tape to ensure it is secured in place. To further secure the polyfill, use duct tape.

This is an important step, and it serves two purposes. The first is it ensures contaminants don't enter the fruiting chamber. The spawn that is fully colonized will be placed in the monotub. This means the mycelium will be mature enough to stand the risk of contamination. The second function it serves is it retains the humidity in the monotub. Fresh air will reach the mycelium without drying out the humidity present within. If you don't cover the holes, the water vapor will evaporate, and the necessary levels of humidity cannot be attained within the fruiting chamber. This, in turn, will obstruct the growing process.

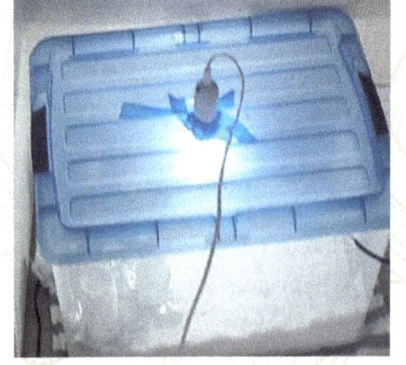

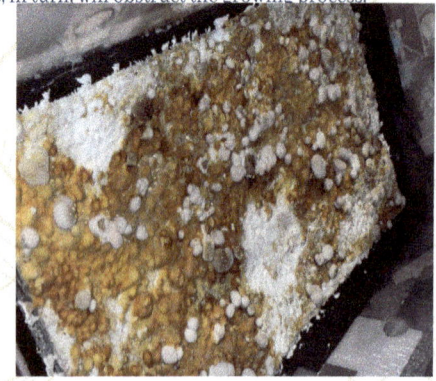

Monotub Fruiting Chambers

The ideal time to harvest mushrooms is before they become too big. Once the caps are fully open, they become prone to contamination. Also, mushrooms start deteriorating rapidly once fully mature. Gently grip the mushroom along the base while gently twisting and pulling it. Harvest the mushroom when they are relatively young, after the first flush. The bed will produce a couple of more flushes until the substrate is fully spent.

If you want the bed to keep producing consecutive harvests, feeding it is essential; this means you will need to keep adding fresh layers of wood chips. However, you don't necessarily have to keep adding more spawns every year. The mycelium from one grow cycle will help reestablish another cycle of mushrooms. Add wood chips to the top of the bed and shuffle it with a rake to mix the chips with existing mycelium in the bed. After this, regularly water the bed for more mushrooms!

Plastic Grow Bag

This is perhaps the easiest means to make a fruiting chamber at home. A filter patch is covered with a large plastic bag that has a hole for ventilation in it. If you don't want to make it at home, you can use a store-bought plastic grow bag as well. As with a monotub, the bottom of the grow bag is lined with a substrate that offers the required humidity for fruiting.

- Materials and Tools Needed
- Large and thick clear plastic bag
- Filter patch
- Glue
- Duct tape
- A pair of scissors

Steps to Follow

The first step is to get a clear plastic bag that is large enough for the yield you want to grow. The larger the bag, the better it is for growing mushrooms. Ideally, it needs to be around 18-inches tall, 8-inches wide, and 5-inches deep. Ensure the bag is sturdy and durable, and it isn't a flimsy trash bag. The ideal plastic bag for making a fruiting chamber should be between 0.2 and 0.5 microns.

Now, use a pair of scissors to cut a hole in the bag. This hole should be large enough to promote sufficient air circulation. At the same time, it should also be small enough that the filter patch can cover it fully. The size of the bag and the filter patches you decide to use will determine the size of the hole. Always ensure the hole is cut along the top part of the bag and is a couple of inches away from the opening.

Using either tape or glue, cover the whole with the filter patch. Ensure the hole is completely covered with the filter. The edges need to be sealed thoroughly, but the filter patch should not be blocked. If it is blocked, this will result in an increased buildup of CO_2 while reducing oxygen available for the mycelium to grow.

Now, the grow bag is complete and ready for use. Simply fill it with the required substrate, inoculate it, and use it to spawn mushrooms of your choice. If you are using them to grow, ensure the bag's bottom is covered with fresh spawn. Once you do this, don't forget to tie up the top part of the grow bag. This creates an air balloon that keeps the bag from collapsing onto itself. At the same time, the filter will ensure that sufficient air is circulating in the bag. However, this might not be sufficient, and therefore, you need to open the bag a couple of times daily and fan it.

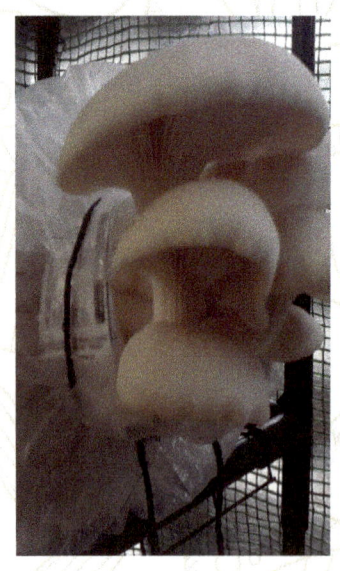

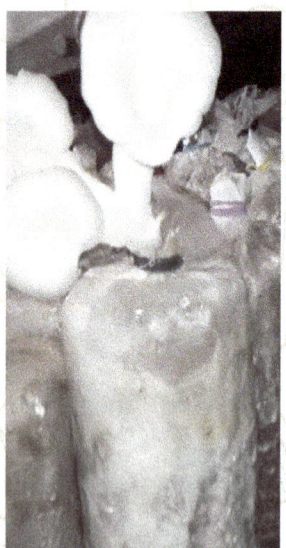

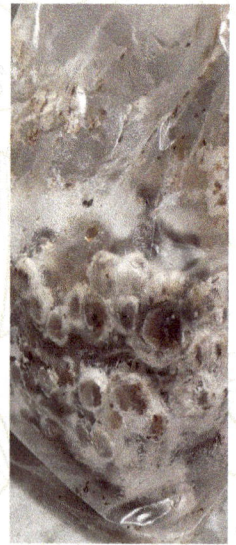

Plastic Grow Bag

4. Mushroom Cultivation Techniques

Mushrooms come in a variety of sizes, shapes, textures, and colors. Due to this variety, the cultivation techniques used for them also vary greatly. Previously, you were introduced to the different considerations to remember while growing mushrooms indoors and outdoors. Now, let's look at all the different cultivation techniques.

1. Grain Spawn

Mushroom spawn is needed for inoculating the substrate regardless of the mushroom you want to grow or the technique you decide to use. You can purchase different types of spawns from the internet or even the local gardening store. That said, it's quite easy to make one at home. While making mushroom spawn, you need a food source for the mycelium to grow on. Grain is the ideal food source. The different types of grains that can be used for making spawns include wheat berries, wild bird seed, brown rice, right, millets, barley, rye, sunflower seeds, and even popcorn. The most popular and commonly used grain is rye, followed by wild bird seed.

While making the spawn, it's vital to maintain proper sterile technique. Regardless of the grains you decide to use; they are all highly susceptible to contamination before colonization. If the grain is contaminated before the mycelium is colonized, the entire batch goes to waste. So, always use a disinfectant such as bleach solution, isopropyl alcohol, or Lysol, wear gloves, and use a glove box.

Different options are available for inoculating the grains as well. A liquid culture available in a syringe is the most ideal and easy way for inoculating. This promotes quick colonization and can be easily injected into the lid, so you don't have to keep opening the jar. You can also use spores, colonized agar, or another jar of spawn that's already available. So, let's see how you can make grain spawn at home.

Materials and Tools Needed

- Grain of your choice
- Spore syringe or liquid culture syringe

- Mason jars with lids
- Gloves
- Bleach solution or Lysol
- 70% isopropyl alcohol
- Polyfill
- Oven mitts
- Power drill with 1/4th inch drill bit
- Glove box
- Pressure cooker
- Bucket
- Lighter or Bunsen burner
- Cooking pot
- A block of wood

Steps to Follow

Preparing the Grain

The first step is to prepare the grain. To do this, you need to select a grain of your choice from the options discussed above. About 3/4th of the sterilized jar must be filled with grain. So, carefully measure grains according to this ratio. Remember, the grains will be cooked, and they will expand once they have absorbed their field capacity of water. If you are using a quart jar filled with dried grain, it will suffice to create spawn for three-quart jars. You can always throw an extra handful to be on the safe side.

Once you have measured the grains, ensure you have rinsed them thoroughly. There shouldn't be any dust, dead insects, crushed grain, or other contaminants on their surface. Simply place the grains in a large strainer and keep them under running water. Move your hands through the grains to clean them. Once the water starts running clear from the grains, it means they are clean.

Now, it's time to soak the grains. The grains need to be soaked for around 12- 24 hours. Ideally, opt for a large pot or a 5-gallon bucket so the grains can stay submerged in water. This step is crucial because certain types of bacteria might survive the sterilization process until they are sprouted. By sprouting the grains, you are reducing the chances of contamination.

Preparing the Jars

Once the grains are in place, let's move on to preparing the jar's lids. First, a hole needs to be cut into the center of the lid used to inoculate the grains using a syringe. This hole also acts as an exhaust that supports the exchange of gases. So, you will need to block it to prevent contaminants from entering the jar and spoiling the spawn. For inoculating grain spawn, you can either purchase lids professionally created for a specific purpose or make it on your own. The simplest way to do it is by drilling a hole in the jar's lid and covering it with polyfill. Carefully drill a hole using the drill bit through the center of the lid. Stuff polyfill into this hole until it is tightly packed. Any excess polyfill can be cut from the top and bottom of the lid.

Cooking the Grains

Once the grains have soaked for 12-24 hours, place them in the strainer. By now, the grains would have almost doubled in size. Before placing them in a large cooking pot, rinse them thoroughly once again. Once the water comes to a boil, cook the grains for 10-15 minutes. Remove the grains from the heat as soon as they pop or crack open. The grains should stay intact because cracked open ones are more susceptible to contamination. When you are cooking the grains, they become soft, making it easier for the mycelium to colonize. The second function is it ensures they cannot absorb more water and have reached their field capacity.

Draining the Grains

Remove the pot from the heat and place the grains in a strainer. Let them dry by spreading them on a flat and clean surface such as a towel or anything absorbable. Let them sit for a couple of hours until they have cooled down and are dry to touch. If you notice there isn't any moisture on the surface, and they are dry to touch, they are ready. Next, you need to check whether the grains are ready for sterilization or not. Ensure the grains should feel soft and fat but are relatively dry on the outside. The grains shouldn't stick together, and you must be able to see the loose kernels.

Filling the Jars Next to Line

Fill the mason jars such that they are 3/4th or 2/3rd full. Some space must be available at the top of the jar for shaking the grains after the sterilization and during the colonization process. Screw the lids on. For additional protection, secure the lids with a square of aluminum foil to reduce additional moisture from entering the jar during colonization.

Sterilization

Now, it's time to pressure-cook the jars to kill any traces of contaminants or living organisms present on the grains. Take the pressure cooker and place a rack on the bottom. This prevents the jar from directly touching the pressure cooker during the cooking process. You can also line the bottom of the pressure cooker with the metal lids or rings of the mason jars. Pour water into the pressure cooker such that there are at least 1- two inches of it at the bottom. Place the loaded jars on top of the rock. After this, simply seal the lid off into the pressure cooker and place it on high heat.

Reduce the heat once the cooker has reached 15 PSI. At this stage, allow it to cook for another 90 minutes before removing it from heat. Before opening the pressure cooker, ensure the pressure levels have returned to the normal ones. Once it is safe, open the pressure cooker using an oven Mitt and remove the jars. Vigorously shake the jars to ensure the grains will not stick. The jars will take up to 8 hours to cool down fully.

Inoculation

Previously, you were introduced to different steps that can be followed for creating a glove box:

- Ensure that you have sterilized the glove box using 10% bleach solution or Lysol.
- Wear the gloves and ensure they have rubbed them down with 70% isopropyl alcohol for further sterilization.
- The jars need to be placed inside the sterilized glove box.

Before putting it inside, ensure you have wiped down the jars with isopropyl alcohol and tissues, so they are thoroughly sterile.

Once you have placed the jars inside, it's time to sterilize your hands once again before inoculating them. Take the syringe and heat it with a lighter or Bunsen burner until it is red hot. Wipe off the needle with an alcohol-soaked towel or a tissue to rapidly cool it down. Inject 2ccs of liquid culture or spore culture into the jar through the polyfill-filled hole at the top. Shake the jar vigorously to ensure the spores in the liquid culture have moved around and entered the grains. Depending on the number of jars you are making, all the steps discussed above need to be repeated.

Colonization

This step is all about patience. The jars need to be removed from the glove box and placed elsewhere for colonization. The area needs to receive sufficient ambient light but shouldn't be exposed to direct sunlight. Maintain an ideal room temperature and ensure it is neither too hot nor cold. While using liquid culture, the first signs of the mycelium can be seen within a few days. On the other hand, while using spores, you'll need to wait for up to two weeks to see the mycelium germinate.

Shake the individual jars vigorously once it has reached about 30% colonization. This speeds up the process of colonization and ensures the mycelium has mixed with the uncolonized areas. Let the jars rest and the grain will be fully colonized within a week.

If you have completed all the steps mentioned until now, the grain spawn is ready for utilization. This can be used with most of the growing techniques discussed in this book except the log grow, PF Tek, and straw logs techniques. By now, you will notice that the spawn in the jars has consolidated to form a single block of mycelium. Using this grain spawn, you'll need to break this block and spread it on a flat surface. Keep the jar covered with something soft such as a towel, as a precautionary measure against accidental breakage.

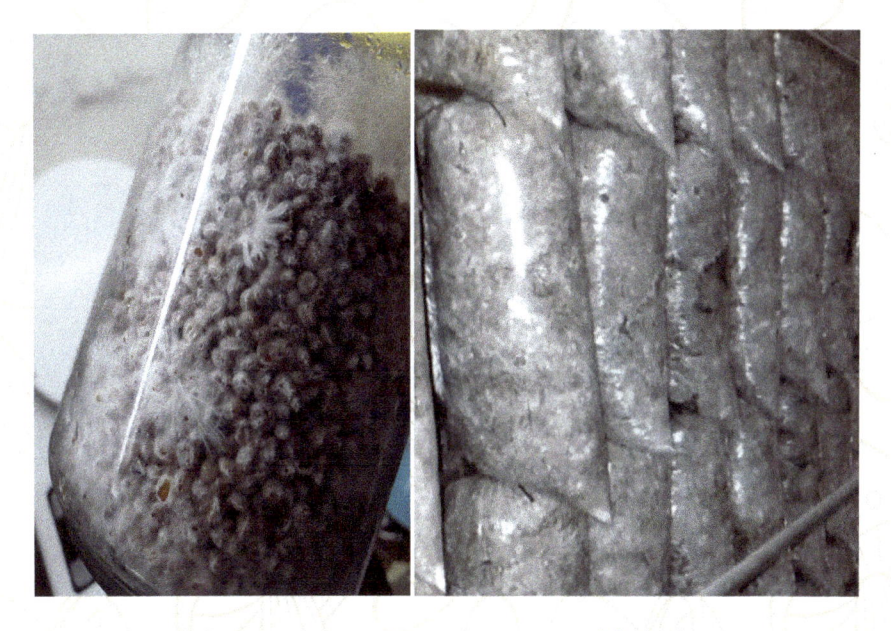

Grain Spawn   Colonization

2. PF Tek

This is an almost foolproof method and is ideal for beginners. It will introduce you to the basics of the mushroom cultivation process. Even though this technique was initially created to cultivate specific psychedelic mushrooms known as psilocybin cubensis, it can be easily used for most species.

This method was developed by Robert McPherson and is popularly known as Psilocybe Fanaticus. This is what the PF in PF Tek stands for!

In this method, the substrate is brown rice flour mixed with vermiculite. The brown rice flour can be substituted with dung, sawdust, or any other material depending on the growing needs of the mushrooms.

Materials and Tools Needed

- Mason jars
- Vermiculite
- A syringe with liquid culture or spores
- Brown rice flour
- Glove box
- 70% isopropyl alcohol
- Micropore tape
- Gloves
- Lighter or Bunsen burner
- Pressure cooker
- Measuring cup
- Power drill
- Mixing bowl
- Shotgun fruiting chamber (with a layer of perlite)
- Steps to Follow
- Preparing the lids

The lids need to be prepared for inoculation. To do this, you will need to drill 2-4 holes on the opposite sides of the lid. The holes must be big enough to accommodate the needle of the syringe. You can use a power drill with a small drill bit attachment. Alternatively, you can also use a hammer and nail to make these holes.

Mixing the Substrate

This method usually uses a combination of vermiculite and brown rice flour as a substrate. Sawdust can also be used instead of flour, depending on the species of mushrooms you are growing. While mixing the vermiculite with sawdust, ensure the ratio of vermiculture to water and brown rice is 2:1:1, respectively. The quantity once again depends on the number of jars you want to prepare. As a rule of thumb, it is better to make a little more than end up with less material. You will need about 4.2 cups of vermiculite and 2.1 cups of water and brown rice flour to make substrate fill six mason jars.

Whenever you mix the substrate, ensure the water and vermiculite must be mixed before combining it with brown rice flour. The substrate must be thoroughly mixed. The final product you end up with will not be sticky and will instead be nice and airy. If the substrate is sticky, something went wrong while combining the ingredients, and you will need to repeat the process.

Filling the Jars

Spoon the substrate carefully into the jars until about half an inch is left at the top of the jar. The substrate shouldn't be sticking to the sides of the jar where you have left the gap. If there is any, ensure you have carefully wiped it, or else it increases the risk of contamination. The substrate shouldn't be compacted and should instead be lightly packed with plenty of air, making it easier for colonization. Dry vermiculite needs to be used for filling the rest of the jar. This shields the contains from further contamination. Place the lids upside down and seal them with aluminum foil to prevent any water from entering the jar during pressure-cooking.

Pressure Cooking

Add water to the pressure cooker such that there are about 1.5-2-inches of water at the bottom. The cooker should be large enough to hold the jars you want to sterilize. The jars should not touch the bottom of the pressure cooker and need to be placed on a rack. The jars prepared in the previous step need to be placed into the pressure cooker. Seal the lid and ensure it is locked in place. Please turn on the heat and let the pressure cooker heat up until it has reached 15 PSI of pressure. Once it has reached this, slightly reduce the heat and let it maintain 15 PSI for up to one hour. Turn off the heat but don't open the pressure cooker lid after this. Let the pressure cooker fully cool down. This process takes up to 8-10 hours. Once you open it, the jars are ready for inoculation.

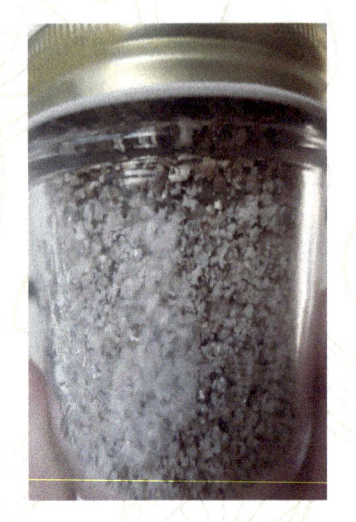

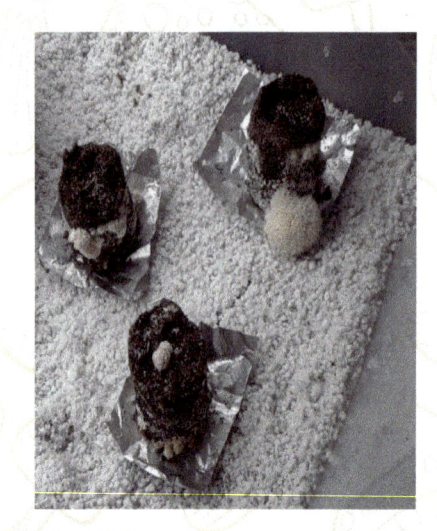

PF Tek: Few days after inoculation

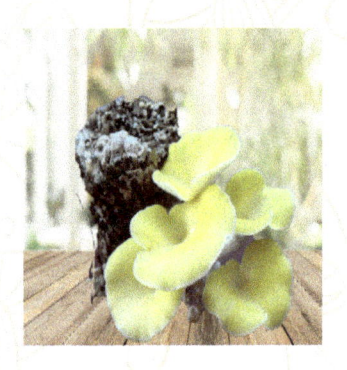

Golden Mushroom through PF Tek   Failed oyester mushroom through PF Tek

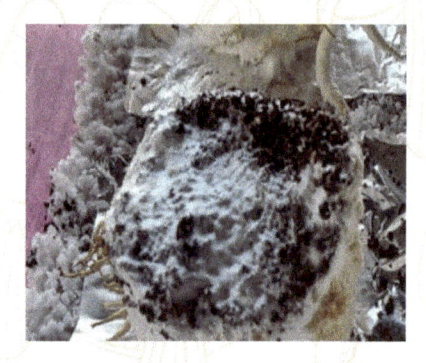

Inoculation

You need to be extra careful during this step. Proper sterile techniques need to be maintained during inoculation. From wearing gloves and using a glove box to sterilizing the syringes between injection points and wiping everything down with rubbing alcohol, be cautious. It's always better to err on the side of caution when it comes to sterilization. Follow the sterilization techniques mentioned in the "Grain Spawn" technique you were introduced to in the previous section.

To get started with the inoculation process, open the pressure cooker and load the jars into the glove box. Before you do this, remove the aluminum foil, wipe down your hands with rubbing alcohol, heat the metal tip of the syringe, and wipe it down with an alcohol wipe. After this, insert the syringe into the first inoculation point created on the lid of the mason jar. Push 0.5cc of the spore or liquid culture into the hole. Always place the needle such that it goes past the layer of dry vermiculture and into the substrate. Repeat this step for all the four holes drilled into the lid.

Colonization

Once the jars are colonized, you need to wait for the mycelium to colonize. For more species of mushrooms, room temperature is ideal for colonization. Cover the inoculation point with micro tape to prevent further contamination while allowing sufficient air to enter the jar. The time required for attaining full colonization depends on the species of mushrooms you are trying to grow and whether you are using spores or liquid culture.

Full colonization can occur anywhere from a few weeks to several months. During this, the jar shouldn't be exposed to direct sunlight and ensure ambient temperature and light are available in the chosen area. Once the jars are fully colonized, they will be completely white. If there are any black or green spots, or any other discoloration, and if the jars have wet and slimy spots, it means they are contaminated. If there is any contamination in the jar, throw it away and don't open it in the area where the others are placed. This prevents further contamination through indirect contact.

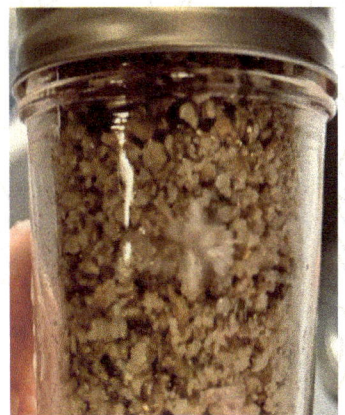

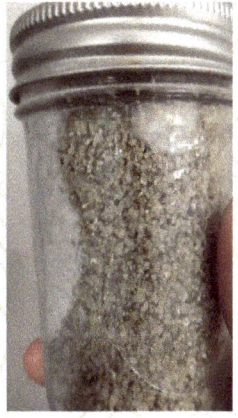

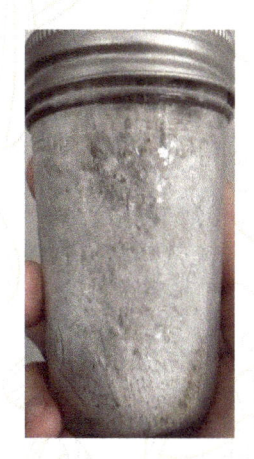

Gradual Colonization

Fruiting Chamber

You need a shotgun fruiting chamber for this technique. The steps to make a fruiting chamber at home were given in the "Growing Mushrooms at Home" chapter in this book. For PF Tek, the bottom of the fruiting chamber must be lined with 3-4-inches of wet perlite.

Dunk And Roll

Now that the fruiting chamber is ready, it's time to birth and rehydrate the colonized cakes. To do this, the cakes need to be submerged in water for up to 24-hours. This process is known as dunking.
Ensure that you place a plate or something heavy on the cakes to keep them submerged or else they will float. After the cakes have soaked for 24-hours, take them out and place them under running water. The colonized cakes are usually resistant to most contaminants and you don't nearly have to be as careful as you were in the previous steps.

Rinse the cakes and roll them in dry vermiculite until they are coated evenly. This is the dunk and roll procedure.

Fruiting

This is the fun part of the cultivation process. The colonized cakes that were dunked and rolled need to be introduced to the fruiting chamber. Once you do this, you simply need to wait for the pins to appear. Take a small square of aluminum foil and place it on the cake such that the cake's bottom does not directly touch the perlite. The aluminum foil needs to separate the cake from perlite but shouldn't cover the entire surface area at the top.

The temperature and humidity level in the chamber must be ideal for the mushroom species you are cultivating. Depending on the species, it will take anywhere between a couple of weeks until a month before you see the pins. Once they appear, the mushrooms start maturing quickly. When they are ready, harvest the fruits and another flush will appear.

You can get up to 3-4 flushes from each colonized cake before it is fully spent. You can also bury the spent cakes in a compost pile to start growing another batch of mushrooms outdoors.

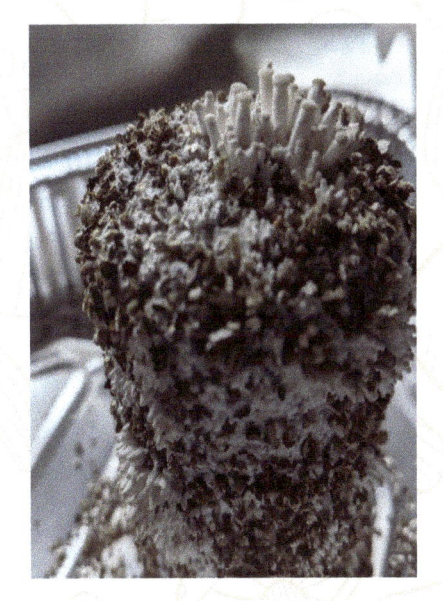

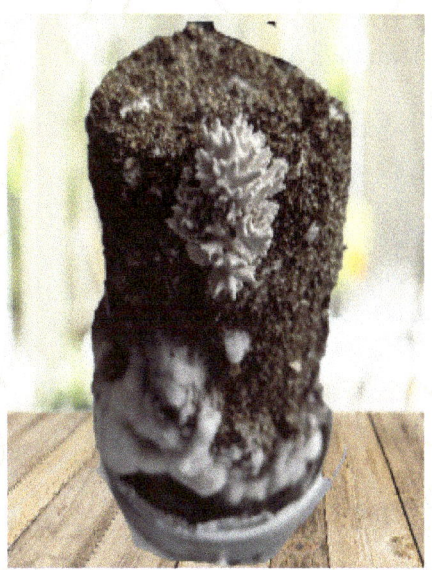

Fruiting

3. 5-Gallon Bucket

It is a simple and easy technique but can be used to grow most varieties of mushrooms.

Almost all the materials and tools needed for this method can be sourced from a local hardware store. Apart from this, the necessary supplies are not expensive for this method.

You can grow different types of mushrooms, but oyster mushrooms thrive while using this method. As mentioned, this is a straightforward technique and can be used for growing high yields at home. The bucket will produce large-sized fruits and in good quantities. If done right, you can get several flushes of yield from a single grow.

Perhaps the only drawback of using this method is it relies excessively on the local climatic conditions. So, if you are living in an arid region, this technique cannot be used. In such instances, an indoor growing technique will come in handy. The buckets should be placed outdoors for fruiting during spring, summer, and fall for ideal results.

Materials And Tools Needed

- Wood chips
- 5-gallon bucket with a lid
- Mushroom spawn
- Large plastic bag
- Large trash bag
- Spray bottle
- Power drill with 1/4th inch drill bit

Steps To Follow

Preparing the Bucket

The first step is to prepare the bucket. As the name mentioned, you'll need a 5-gallon bucket. Start by drilling holes in it. The holes drilled will be used as outlets for the mushrooms during the fruiting phase. So, ensure the holes are around 1/4th-inch wide for this method. You can also make the holes about 1/2 to 3/4th-inch wide. Don't believe that the larger holders make bigger fruit. Unfortunately, this usually means the substrate will dry out quickly due to large holes.

You need to drill holes all around the bucket. Each hole needs to be 2-3 inches apart from one another. Towards the bottom of the bucket, you can add some smaller holes that allow all the excess water to drain. For instance, if the normal holes are 1/4th-inch wide, the smaller holes can be about 1/8th-inch.

Pasteurizing the Substrate

Now, it is time to pasteurize the substrate. Depending on the species you are trying to grow, the substrate will differ. That said, the most common ones used for the 5-gallon method are straw or wood chips. The simplest way to pasteurize the substrate is by placing the wood chips in a large plastic tote. You can either use a plastic tote bag or any other plastic bag that can withstand high temperatures. After this, you need to fill it with hot water. The ideal temperature needs to be between 150-180°F to ensure all the contaminants are eliminated during pasteurization. If the water is not hot enough, this step will become meaningless.

After this, leave the wood chips to soak in water for up to 8 hours. Please don't remove them from the bag until they have cooled down to room temperature.

Getting Ready For Inoculation

Now that you have pasteurized the wood chips, it's time for inoculation. Please ensure the wood chips are cool to touch. If the substrate is too hot, the mycelium will be killed upon contact. The wood chips should be hydrated but shouldn't be dripping wet. As mentioned in the previous methods, the substrate is highly damp or moist, which increases the risk of contamination later. Over hydrated substrate becomes a hotspot for bacterial contamination. If the substrate seems to be over hydrated, squeeze out the excess water from it.

Adding the Spawn

Now, it is time to start adding the spawn and wood chips to the bucket. Start by layering the bucket with a substrate that's about 1.5 inches thick. On this layer, place a layer of mushroom spawn. After this, layer it with wood chips and then add another layer of spawn. Keep doing this until you reach the top. Ensure that the first layer visible in the bucket is made of the substrate and not the spawn. If the spawn is directly exposed to external elements, the mycelium will not grow, and instead, the risk of contamination increases. You will need more wood chips than spawn. Generally, about 90% of the bucket will be covered with substrate and the rest with spawn. Typically, a 5-gallon bucket will need about 2-2.5 lbs of spawn.

Colonization

Once you have layered the bucket like lasagna, it's time to put the lid on the bucket. Now you simply need to wait for the spawn to colonize. During this phase, place the bucket in a darkened and cool space away from direct sunlight. The best place to do this would be in the basement or the garage. Ensure the ambient temperature is not hot. If you are living in an apartment, place the bucket in a closet and it will do the trick. As long as you keep it out of direct sunlight, it is all good.

Another consideration during this step is to ensure the substrate doesn't dry out too much. If this happens, the mycelium will die too. To avoid this:

- Drape some plastic over the bucket.
- Don't wrap it tightly; and instead, give it some breathing space.
- Leave the bucket undisturbed for a week.
- After seven days, open the bucket to see the progress.
- Dig into the top layer of wood chips, and you can see mycelial growth. You will also notice a pleasant smell of mushrooms.

If something smells bad or stinks, it's a sign of contamination. If you believe the bucket has any contaminants in it, you should get rid of it immediately, sanitize the entire area before starting again.

Depending on the mushrooms you are growing and the temperature it is exposed to, full colonization can take anywhere between 10-21 days.

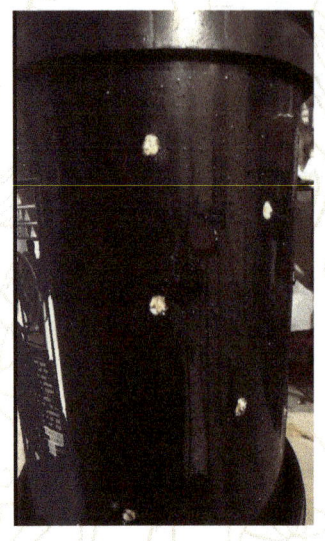

Preparing Bucket

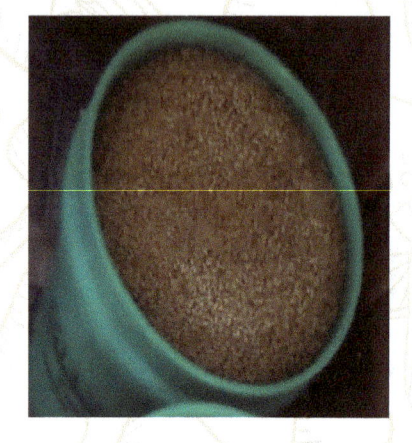

Making Grain Spawn

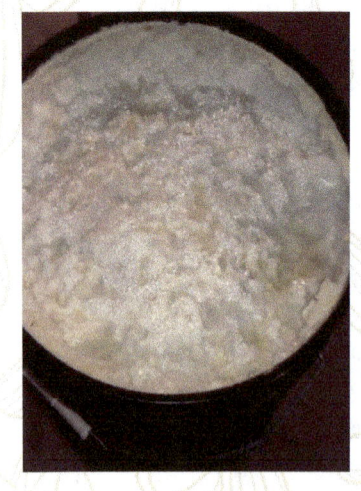

Post Inoculation

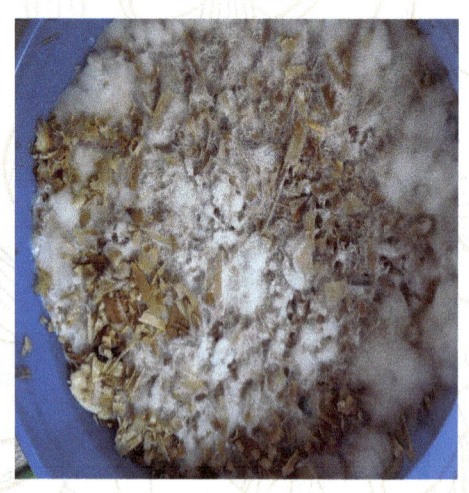

Colonization

Fruiting

Once the bucket is fully colonized, it's time for fruiting. While fruiting, you will need to place the bucket in an area that receives sufficient light for at least twelve hours daily. If natural light cannot suffice this requirement, you can use artificial lights as well. That said, the bucket should also stay in the dark for the next twelve hours. If the climatic conditions seem appropriate, this bucket can also be placed outdoors during the fruiting stage. Even when it is kept outdoors, ensure it is not directly exposed to sunlight. It needs to be placed in the shade.

Fruiting will be visible within a week if everything goes right. The pins will start appearing in small clusters through the holes you drilled into the bucket. That said, the fruiting period also varies depending on the species and climatic conditions. Ensure the pins do not dry out at this stage. If this happens, all your efforts until now will have gone to waste. If you are placing the bucket outdoors ensure it is not too windy, dry and hot, or cold because the pins are quite fragile. You can loosely drape a plastic sheet around the bucket to protect them from harsh elements.

Once the pins have appeared, the maturation process will take place within no time. The fruits would be full-sized and ready for harvest within 10 days since the first pins appeared.

Harvesting

The best time to have mushrooms is once they are fully formed and their caps have expanded. Try to harvest the mushrooms before they start dropping their spores. Harvesting them early is always better than harvesting late. If you harvest too late, their texture and taste will be significantly altered. Whenever you are harvesting, make sure that you are pulling the mushrooms in clumps and try to get them as close to the base as you possibly can. Try to leave the mycelium undisturbed to promote future growth.

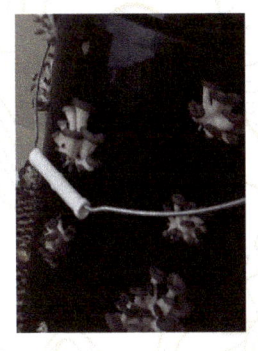

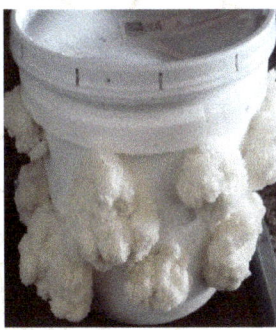

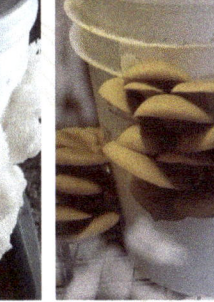

Fruiting   Ready to Harvest

4. Monotub Grow Method

If you are interested in obtaining significant yields without growing outdoors and want to use a small space inside your home, a monotub will come in handy. All you need is a large plastic storage bin and you can produce multiple flushes of different varieties of edible mushrooms at home. The monotub is fashioned from a large container.

So, the space you opt for needs to be big enough to accommodate this container. A basement, garage, or even a closet, can be used for cultivating mushrooms. While using a monotub, especially while cultivating at home, is easier when you are starting from colonized mushroom spawn

While using this method, there won't be any exchange of fresh air. This might become problematic for the mycelium of certain species of mushrooms. For instance, oyster mushrooms require a little fresh air while growing.

That said, the monotub can be rigged to ensure the free flow of air fill. You simply need to attach a small computer fan to the fruiting chamber for maximizing airflow. If this seems like too much work, simply fan the container a couple of times daily.

Even if the fruits look smaller or slightly deformed, their taste will not be compromised while growing them using a monotub.

Materials and Tools Needed

- Mason jars with lids (quart-sized)
- Mushroom spawn
- Sufficient substrate
- Spray bottle
- 70% isopropyl alcohol
- Large pot
- Monotub fruiting chamber

Steps to Follow

Hydrating the Substrate

You will need to hydrate the substrate. In this method, you will be using a significant amount of substrate because you will have to fill up a 70-quart container with it. Therefore, the bulk substrate needs to be hydrated. To do this, gradually water the substrate. Don't add too much water at once because overhydration increases the risk of contamination. To hydrate the substrate, keep adding a little water to it and check regularly. To do this, pick up the substrate and squeeze it.

If water drips only when you squeeze it and not while holding it, it has reached its field capacity. At this stage, stop watering it. You don't have to check the entire substrate. Instead, test a random handful, and this will do.

Pasteurization

Now, it's time to pasteurize the bulk substrate. Start by filling quart-sized mason jars with the substrate you have hydrated in the previous step.

Depending on the size of the monotub, the number of jars required for pasteurization will also differ. Usually, about 8-10 quart-sized mason jars with lids will be sufficient for a 70-quart monotub.

Fill the jars with the substrate without tightly screwing on the lids. If you seal them at this stage, opening them later will become extremely difficult. Next, place the jars in the large pot and ensure the water in it has come to a level that's right below the jar's lid.

Next, put the pot on the stove and let the water heat to 160-180°F. Use a candy thermometer to maintain this temperature range. Let the jars stay in the pot for another hour before turning off the heat. Let the jars cool down naturally before moving to the next step.

This can take up to 8 hours, so be patient. The jars need to be cold to touch when you remove them from the pot. If they are still hot, the mycelium will die upon contact.

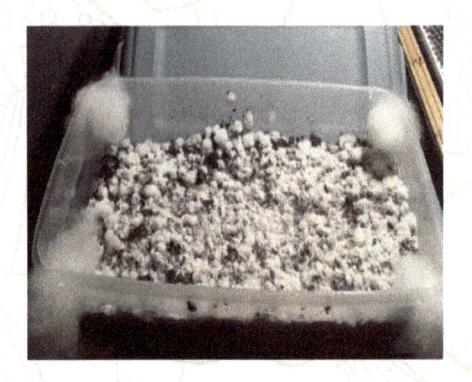

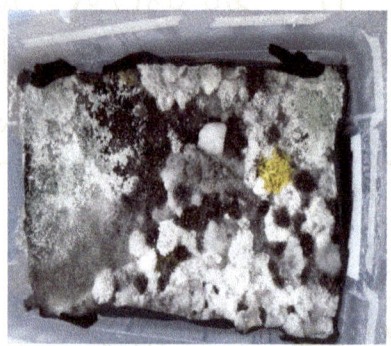

Monotub Colonization

Sterilization

The monotub needs to be sterilized before you can add spawn and substrate to it. This is quite a simple step. You can either put a 10% bleach solution or 70% isopropyl alcohol in a spray bottle. Spray the solution on the inside of the monotub. Then, carefully wipe down all the surfaces using a rag or paper towels.

Layering the Monotub

Now that the monotub is sterilized, it's time to layer the substrate and spawn. At this stage, the bulk substrate should have returned to room temperature.

Remove it from water and ensure the jars are always cold to touch. Open the jar and sprinkle the substrate along the bottom of the monotub. Each layer of substrate needs to be about an inch thick. After this, add a layer of spawn that's about half an inch thick.

Top it with another layer of bulk substrate and spawn. Keep going until you have created lasagna-like layers that are about 3-5 inches thick. The top layer should always be of the substrate and not the spawn.

Colonization

Now, place the monotub in a dark place for colonization. Ensure that it is never exposed to direct sunlight and instead receives a little ambient light.

It doesn't need any specific temperature, and room temperature will be fine. As long as the weather doesn't get too hot or cold, the mycelium will grow. You will start seeing the white spots of the mycelium appear across the top layer of the substrate within ten days. The entire monotub should be colonized within a few weeks. When it is completely colonized, the top layer of the substrate will be covered with thin mycelium. If you notice any funky smells, discoloration, or unnatural wet spots, the batch has been contaminated, and you will have to start again.

Fruiting

Once the monotub is fully colonized, it is ready for fruiting. To kickstart the fruiting process, place a trash bag over the monotub such that the top layer filled with mycelium is fully covered.

Depending on the species and the growing conditions, pins will appear within a couple of days or a few weeks. Once the pins appear, the mushrooms will mature within no time.

Harvesting

Depending on the type of mushrooms you are growing, the harvesting technique will also vary. Some of them can be pulled from the base, while others need to be plucked as close to the base as possible.

You can also cut them using a sharp blade. As mentioned, when using this method of mushroom cultivation, you can obtain multiple flushes from the same monotub after the first harvest. You can get up to 3 flushes, and in some cases, it can even produce seven flushes.

All of this depends on the quality of the substrate you are using and the colonization that's taken place. That said, every subsequent flush will be smaller than the previous one. So, if the first flush itself is not big enough, it's better to start again instead of waiting for prolonged periods for a disappointing yield.

If the moisture level starts running low or the mycelium has weakened, it becomes more vulnerable to different forms of contamination. If you are waiting for the tub to give you multiple flushes, pay close attention to any discoloration or other signs of mold after the first flush. As soon as you see any sign of contamination, the best thing you can do is get rid of the batch altogether and start afresh.

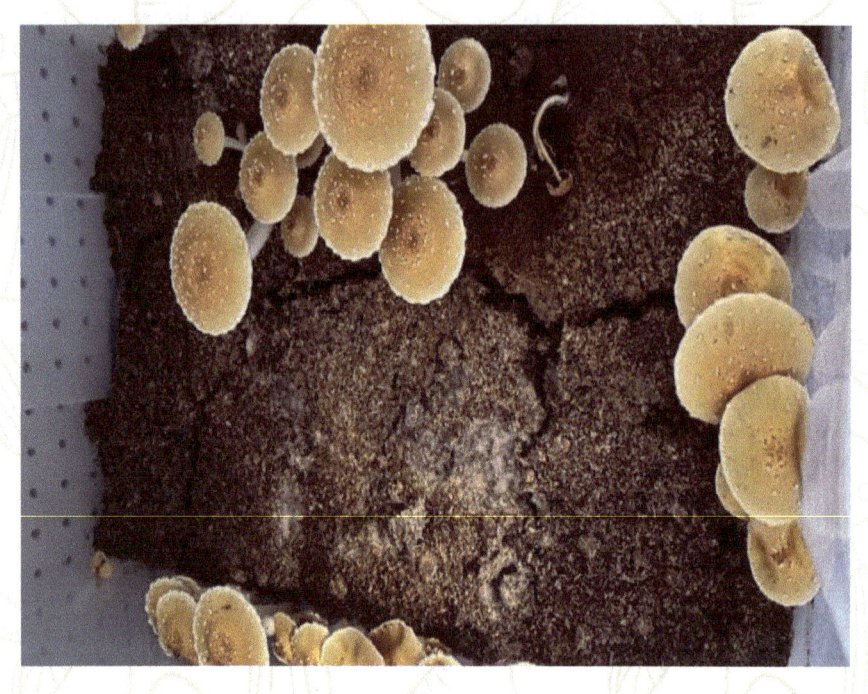

Monotub Fruiting

5. Log Grow Technique

When compared to the other techniques mentioned in this chapter, this is relatively more complex. That said, it also comes with a variety of advantages that others don't offer.

The most important benefit of this technique is that it helps replicate the natural way most fungi grow. Whether it is shiitake and oyster mushrooms or maitake and lion's mane, they all grow on decaying logs in the wild. So when you grow such species on logs, you are replicating the ideal conditions their mycelium needs to grow and thrive.

While using a log to grow mushrooms, the substrate and fruiting chamber will be the log itself. To kickstart the growth of mycelium, you need to add the spawning plugs. If you are living in any wooded areas, you can source the logs from local trees. Most species of mushrooms usually favor hardwood logs. Oyster mushrooms prefer white birch and beech, white oak and maple work well for shiitake mushrooms. The most commonly used logs for cultivating mushrooms are maple, alder, aspen, elm, oak, birch, balsam, and willow.

The only drawback of using this method when compared to others is the time taken for the mycelium to take root. The colonization and fruiting stages will be extended while using the log grow method. After the first flush, you will receive one flush annually for up to six years from the same log before it needs to be replaced.

Whenever you select a log for this technique, make sure that you opt for a healthy one and not a decaying one. If the log is already rotting, the chances of the fungi you are trying to grow competing with undesirable fungi increases. If the log is large, the colonization and fruiting process will take longer. If you are just getting started, start with a small hardwood log about 10-inches long and up to 4-inches wide.

Materials and Tools Needed

- Hardwood log (beech, alder, maple, aspen, balsam, willow, oak, birch, and poplar)
- Spawn plug
- Power drill with 5/16th inch drill bit
- Hammer
- Crockpot, fryer, or an old pot
- Cheese wax

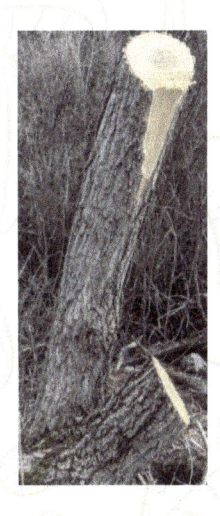

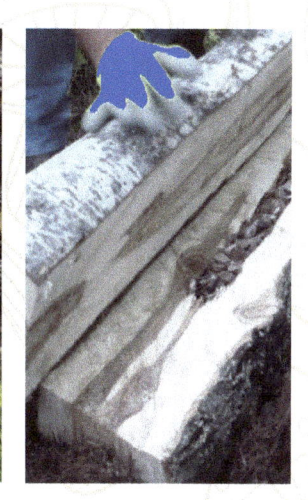

Selecting Logs   Putting Moisture on Logs   Inoculation

Steps to Follow

Selecting a Log

The first thing you need to do is find the right log for the species you are trying to grow. As mentioned, most hardwood logs are an ideal choice for mushrooms. Please be careful while selecting the log because this determines the quality of the flush or yield you will receive. If the log looks like it is rotting or decaying, stay away from it and instead opt for a healthy one. Ideally, opt for logs that were cut down from a tree within the last month or so.

You will need to make a note of the type of wood you are using and its size along with the strain of mushrooms used for colonizing it. All this information will come in handy while making a note of possible combinations that can be used for growing mushrooms in the future.

Drilling Holes

In this method, you'll need to drill several holes in the log for growing mushrooms. In the wild, they grow on their own. Since you are replicating the required conditions, you will need to create some holes in the log. Before you start drilling aimlessly, you will need to figure out the number of holes that will be needed. Every hole that you drill will be filled with a spawn plug.

If you are using a log that's about 3-4 feet long, you will need about 30-50 spawn plugs.

The number of holes you will need to drill can be calculated using this formula:

[Length of the log (in cm) X Diameter of the log (in cm)]/ 60

Now, it is time to start drilling holes along the length of the log. While drilling, use a 5/16th inch drill bit. Ensure the holes are about 6-inches apart along the length of the log. Avoid drilling holes in the top and bottom 2-inches of the log.

The holes drilled need to be 1-inch deep to accommodate the spawn plugs. Once you have drilled the first row of holes, the next row needs to be 2.5-inches apart. Try to position the holes in a staggered fashion. This eventually means the whole should resemble a checkerboard when complete.

Using Spawn Plugs

The spawn plugs will need to be placed into the drilled holes. Gently push the plugs far enough into the whole so they stay in place. To ensure they don't move or come out, gently hammer them. Make sure that you don't use too much force because the plugs can break at this stage. The plug should be placed such that they are below the bark of the wood. When this happens, the flush will appear on the outer side of the upper surface of the log. This also protects the spawn during the inoculation phase.

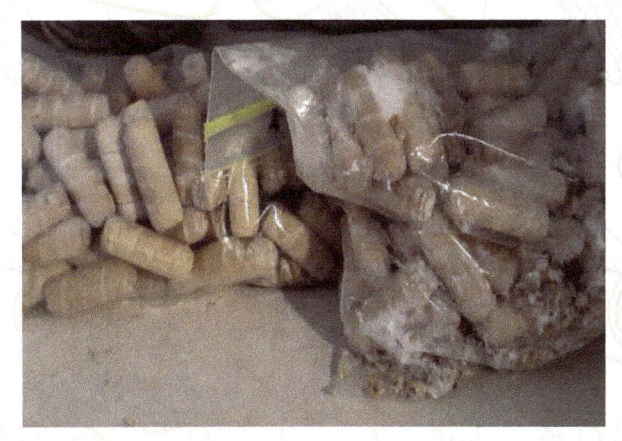

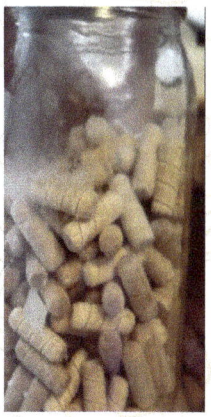

Spawn Plugs

Stealing the Holes

Once you have filled all the holes with spawn plugs, it is time to seal them. When you do this, it ensures contaminants from the external environment do not harm the spawn during colonization. The ideal sealing material is cheese wax. You can use candle wax or beeswax as well, but cheese wax is the preferred option.

To get started with the sealing process, start by melting the wax. You can use a crockpot or even a deep fryer for melting the wax. This will be a slightly messy process and difficult to clean and therefore, the appliance used for melting should be something that you don't mind getting dirty. You will need cotton balls, an old rag, a brush, a cloth, or a wax dabber for applying the melted wax into the openings. Ensure the holes are covered with a thin layer of melted wax to seal them completely from the outside environment.

This seal ensures mold and other fungal spores don't enter the jar through the hole during the colonization phase. It also prevents insects and other critters from eating away the mycelium. Apart from this, this ensures the spawn does not dry out during colonization and fruiting.

Storing the Log

As mentioned, the inoculation stage is quite lengthy in this process. So, be prepared to store the logs for quite some time. They will need to be stored in shade away from direct sunlight. You can place them under a tree, behind bushes, or any other place that gets sufficient shade and is not exposed to direct sunlight. Covering the logs with a shade cloth also reduces their exposure to direct sunlight.

Care During Inoculation

The mycelium will die if the logs dry during incubation. To prevent the logs from drying out completely, they will need to be hosed or watered once or twice a week depending on the climatic conditions of the area you reside. Ensure that you spray the logs for up to 10 minutes every time you water. This helps the logs retain the required level of moisture.

Fruiting

If you are not really patient and want to start seeing the logs fruit early you can initiate early fruiting in this technique. If you don't want to do this, please skip this step and wait patiently until the fruits appear. Usually, fruits take up to 2-3 years to appear in this method. By initiating early fruiting, you can start producing fruits within 6 months.

To do this, you will need to shock the mycelium present in the colonized log. You will need to wait for up to 6-9 months after inoculating them. To shock the log, you need to let it soak in cold water for 24-hours. Once this is done, simply remove the log and wait for the fruits to appear.

Harvesting

If the log is fully colonized it can fruit up to three times within a year. The usual time during which this happens is fall or spring. This can also happen after heavy rains. Once the log is rotting, don't forget to check it frequently. As with all mushrooms, the maturation process is quite quick once the pins appear. Don't forget to harvest mushrooms when they are young instead of waiting for them to fully mature.

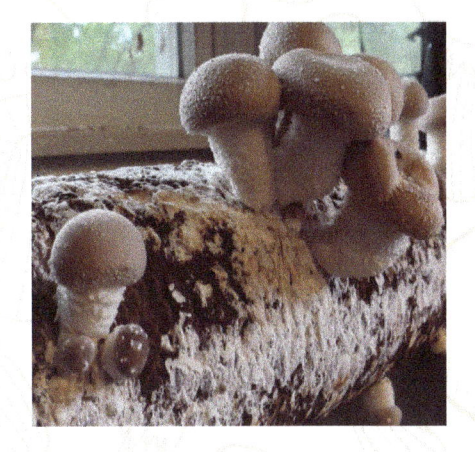

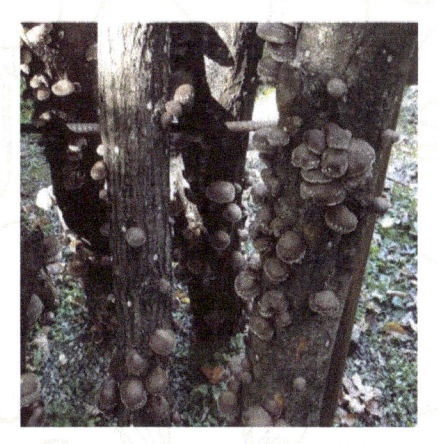

Fruiting

6. Bottle or Jar Grows

You can also start growing mushrooms using mason jars or any bottles with wide mouths. This is not a labor-intensive process and is fairly easy making it ideal for beginners.

One of the most important advantages of using this method is that the materials can be reused. This not only reduces the overall costs involved in cultivation but reduces wastage as well. Harvesting mushrooms also becomes easy when using this method. Apart from it, it's aesthetically pleasing too!

Perhaps the biggest drawback is the mushrooms grown using this technique tend to be smaller in size when compared to other methods.

When mushrooms have a larger environment for fruitings, such as the ones provided by outdoor beds or monotub, the flushes are larger and the fruits are bigger. The relatively small surface area means relatively small flushes. Also, this method produces only a single flush from the substrate and spawn. You will not be using a lot of substrates and therefore, the mycelium will not have sufficient food source for producing multiple flushes associated with other techniques. Even if a second flush appears, it will be quite smaller than the first one.

The most common mushrooms you can grow using this method include enoki, beech, shiitake, maitake, and nameko. The ideal jar or bottle for this method is a quart-sized Mason jar.

Colonized Jar

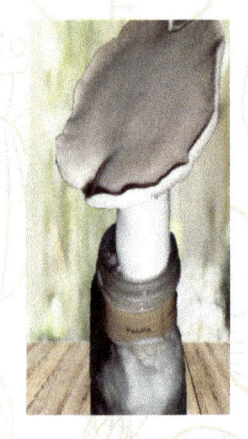

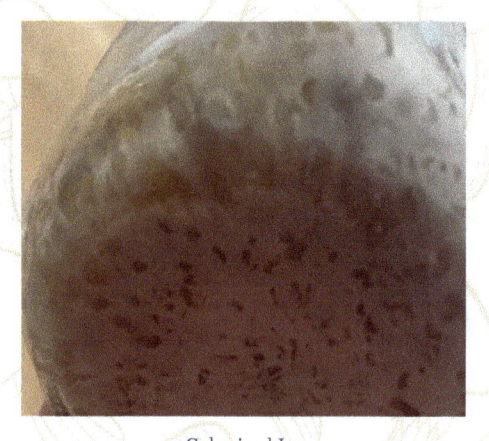

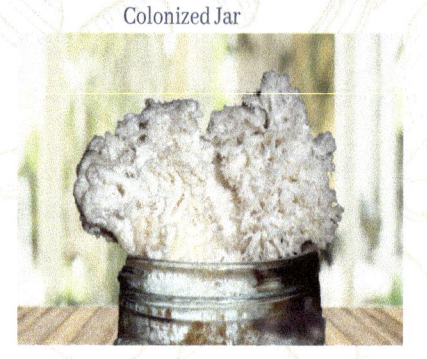

Nameko in a Jar Lion's Mane in a Jar

Materials and Tools Needed

- Mason jars (quart-sized with lids)
- A substrate of your choice
- Mushroom spawn
- Polyfill
- Aluminum foil
- Plastic bowl
- Gloves
- 70% Isopropyl alcohol
- Power drill with 1/4th inch drill bit
- Pressure cooker
- Glove box
- Shotgun fruiting chamber (with a layer of perlite)

Steps to Follow

Preparing the Lids

Before you can use this technique to start growing mushrooms, you need to prepare the lids. The lids need to be altered a little so fresh air can enter the jar without letting any external contaminants enter it.

To do this you will need to drill a 1/4th inch hole in the center of the lid.

Depending on the number of jars you are using, you need to drill a hole in all the lids.

Take some polyfill and push a wad of it through the drilled hole so it tightly secures the space. Any excess polyfill that hangs from the top and bottom of the lids can be cut off using a pair of scissors. This acts as a filter that prevents contaminants from entering the jar without restricting airflow.

Preparing the Substrate

Now, depending on the type of mushrooms you are growing, the chosen substrate will need to be hydrated. The most common substrates used in this cultivation technique are hardwood sawdust that's mixed with soy hulls or wheat bran. The substrate needs to be placed in a large bowl or a container and soaked in water. The substrate shouldn't be too wet and should have reached its maximum field capacity. The hydrated substrate should be filled into the jars. The jars don't have to be tightly packed with the substrate. If the jars are tightly packed, the mycelium cannot colonize easily. Gently tap the jar against a hard surface to ensure the substrate is lightly packed. Fill the jars until about half an inch of space is left at the top.

Creating a Hole in the Substrate

You will need to create a hole in the substrate for pouring the colonized spawn. You simply need to take a long wooden spoon or anything similar to it and push it through the center of the jar until it hits the bottom. This hole should be up to 3/4th inch wide. Once you have created such holes in all the jars, seal the jar with the lid, and then place a piece of aluminum foil on it to cover it further.

Sterilization

Each of the jars needs to be sterilized thoroughly to ensure no mold or bacterial contaminants are present in it. Place a rag or a dishtowel along the bottom of a pressure cooker and place the jar on this. Ensure the jar is never in direct contact with the metal base of the pressure cooker because it can crack during the cooking process. Add water to the pressure cooker such that there is about an inch of water at the bottom. The jars need to be placed in the pressure cooker in an upright position. Place the cooker on the stove, turn on the heat, and wait until it reaches 15 PSI. Once it reaches this pressure, reduce the heat and let it stay for up to 90 minutes. After this, turn off the heat and let the jars cool down within the pressure cooker. This process can take up to eight hours. Don't open the cooker until it has completely cooled down.

Inoculation

Now open the pressure cooker slowly and take the jars out. The jars need to be cool to touch. If not, the heat from it will kill the mycelium. You will need to use a glove box for this step. Start by sterilizing the glove box and quickly move the jars from the pressure cooker into the glove box. Quickly open the jar, pour the spawn directly into the whole you created during the previous step. Ensure you do this as quickly as you possibly can and replace the lid as well. The longer you leave the jar open, the greater the risk of contamination. Repeat this process with all the jars and don't forget to sterilize the glove box between each use.

Colonization

Once you have inoculated all the jars, you simply need to wait for colonization. The jars that are removed from the glove box need to be placed somewhere away from direct light for colonization. The jars can be left at room temperature provided it isn't too hot or cold. Depending on the species and the room temperature, the colonization stage will vary. Usually, in this method, you should see colonization within a month.

Fruiting

The jars need to be introduced into the fruiting chamber once it has fully colonized. To do this, you need to open the jar and use a clean fork to mix the topmost layer of mycelium lightly. After this, replace the jar on the perlite within the fruiting chamber. Don't remove the lids while placing them in the fruiting chamber. The pins should start appearing within a week, and they will develop into full-sized fruits within a couple of days.

Harvesting

It is time to harvest once you have patiently gone through all the steps discussed in this section. You don't have to worry about disturbing the mycelium while using this technique because you usually don't get more than one flush from a single jar.

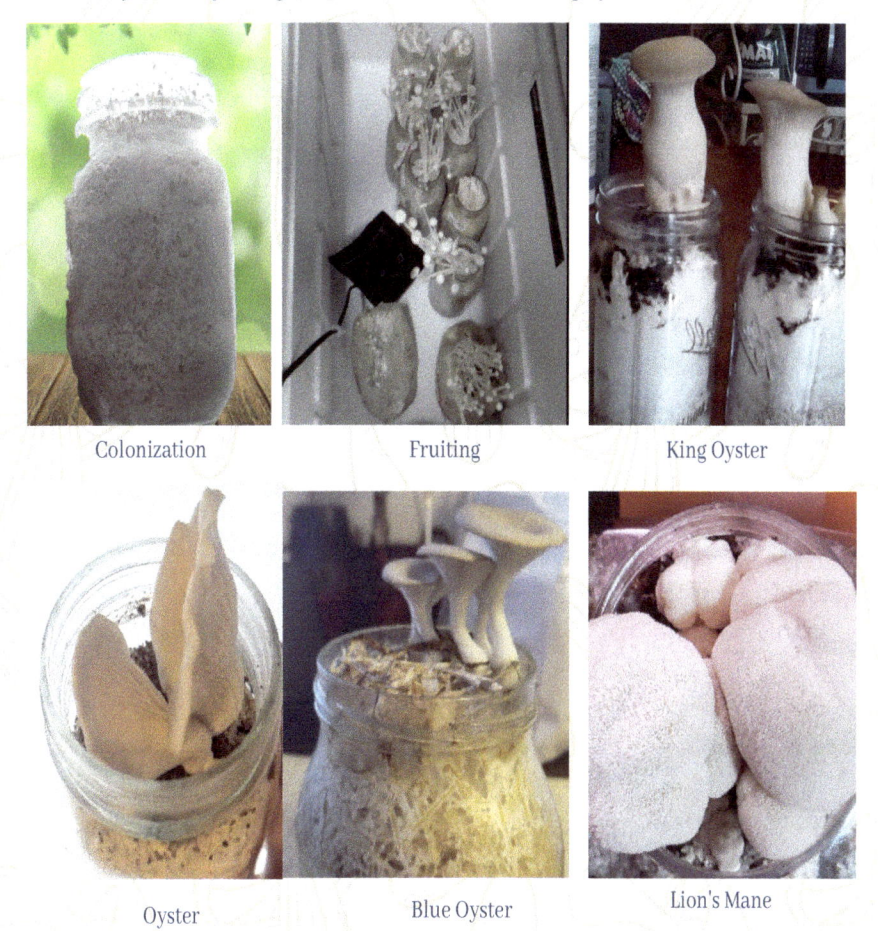

Colonization

Fruiting

King Oyster

Oyster

Blue Oyster

Lion's Mane

Growing Outdoors (Straw Logs)

Growing mushrooms outdoors is quite exciting. One of the benefits is that indoor growing chambers don't provide sufficient oxygen flow, which can be easily circumvented by growing them outdoors in mushroom beds. It not only offers better yields, but the mushrooms will also be bigger, and their appearance can be different too.

For example, King oyster and reishi mushrooms look quite different when exposed to sunlight and an outdoor environment. Depending on the species of mushrooms you want to grow, consider using an outdoor bed.

Creating a bed outdoors is not only easy, but it hardly requires any maintenance. You don't have to worry too much about keeping things as sterile and clean as you need to while growing indoors. On the downside, the bed is usually exposed to all elements. That means you will need to be extra vigilant about tackling pests and other critters from harming the bed.

Materials and Tools Needed

- Oat or wheat straw, (or a colonized straw log)
- Mushroom spawn
- Pillowcase
- Gloves
- 70% isopropyl alcohol
- Large container for pasteurization
- Peat moss
- Garden soil
- 16-inch poly tubing or plastic bag
- Trimmer for chopping straw
- Shovel
- Candy thermometer
- Zip tie

Steps to Follow :

Chopping the Straw

The straw that you have obtained needs to be chopped into smaller pieces.

You can use gardening shears or a string trimmer. The chopped straw needs to be about 1-3-inches long. Each piece doesn't have to be precise as long as they're chopped up evenly. Soak the straw for a couple of hours with a little dish soap. After soaking, don't forget to thoroughly wash it as well.

Pasteurizing

This is quite a simple step. Stuff the draw into a large pillowcase. Place this pillowcase in a large plastic container and fill it with hot water. To keep the pillowcase submerged, you need to place something heavy on it. The water in the container needs to be at about 160°F. Let the pillowcase stay submerged for two hours. If the temperature of water reduces, you can add more hot water. It needs to stay at a constant 160°F. Use a thermometer to check the temperature. After this, let the water come to room temperature naturally before removing the pillowcase. Leave the pillowcase out until all the excess water present in it drains away.

Mixing Spawn and Straw

Now, you will have to inoculate the straw. To do this, add the grain spawn. The pasteurized straw needs to be placed into a plastic container. Before you do this quickly wipe down the container with isopropyl alcohol or bleach solution. You will need to mix the straw and spawn such that you are using 15% spawn and 85% straw. Always use gloves while mixing them with your hands. Do not mix the spawn until the straw has completely cooled down.

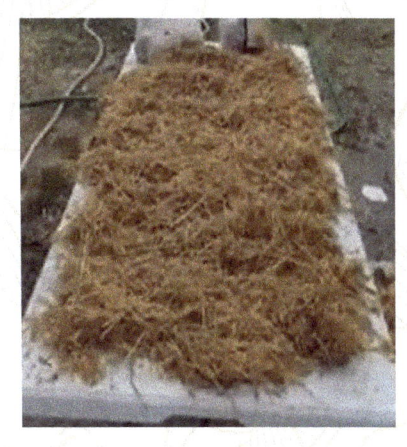

Pasteurizing   Mixing Spawn and Straw

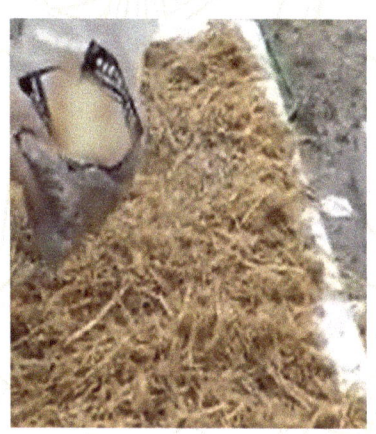

Start Stuffing

You will need to create logs once the straw and substrate are properly mixed. The inoculated straw needs to be stuffed into polytubes or long plastic bags such as a clear trash bag. While using polytubes, ensure the roll is about 16-inches in diameter. The trash bag should also have a similar diameter. Zip tie one end of the bag b before you start stuffing the inoculated substrate into it. Once again, you will need to wear clean gloves while doing this. Pack the substrate tightly into the bag or tube to avoid any air pockets. Do this until you have a log of the desired length. Usually, aim for a log that is about 2-4-inches long. Once you have added sufficient substrate, you will need to twist the top of the bag or the tubing as tightly as you possibly can. Tie the open-end using zip ties. Repeat this process with as many tubes as you need.

Once the tubes are ready, slash X marks into them such that they are 5-inches apart and cover the entire bag. This gives the mycelium sufficient air to grow.

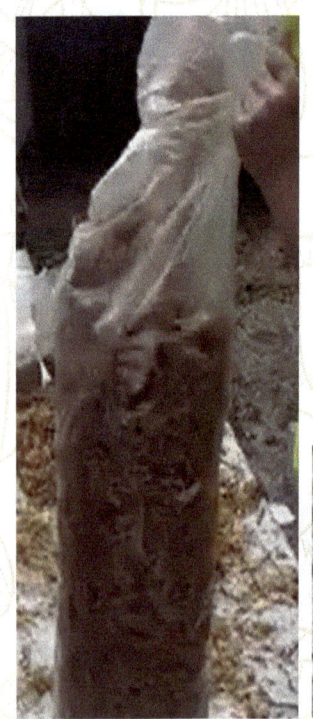

Colonization

Now, you simply need to wait for the colonization to start. During this period, don't place the stuffed bags outdoors. Instead, keep them away from direct sunlight.

The entire colonization should be complete within 1-4 weeks in this method. Don't forget to check on the bags daily. Check for any signs of contamination. If a bag is contaminated, discard it. Once your logs are fully colonized, shift them to the outdoor bed.

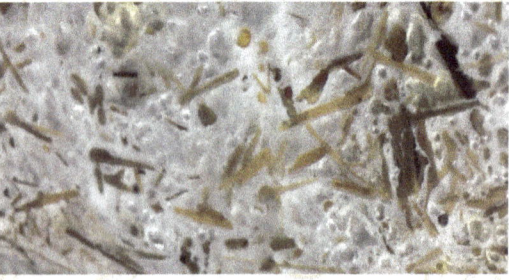

Stuffing

Colonization

Making the Outdoor Bed

You need to create an outdoor bed for the mushrooms you want to grow. Start by selecting the ideal spot. The area shouldn't receive too much direct sunlight. Ideally, look for a shady spot under a tree, or even the side of the house. Ensure the bed you create is big enough to accommodate your colonized logs.

Using Colonized Logs

You will need to cut the colonized logs into disks and then cover them with a casing. The colonized logs need to be cut into disks that are about 2-3 inches thick. You don't have to be too precise while doing this. If the log has started developing fruits, ensure that you remove all the mushrooms and pins from it right now. You can also break the disks in half to create flat edges for the bed.

You will need to make a casing for these disks. The casing layer should be made of a material that doesn't offer any nutritional value whatsoever. So, the ideal layer would be made of equal portions of peat moss and garden soil.

This ensures the bed stays moist and prevents the disks from drying out. Place the soil and peat moss in a large container and mix them thoroughly. Add water to the casing layer until it has reached its field capacity. Just pick up a handful of this mixture and squeeze. If water pours out only when you squeeze it and not when you are holding it, it means it has reached its field capacity.

Maintaining Outdoors Bed

You will need to ensure the outdoor bed stays moist and doesn't dry out. If this happens, the mycelium will die. Ideally, you will need to water the bed daily or on alternate days. This depends on the existing climatic conditions. If the bed looks like it's drying out, water it. On the other hand, if only the top layer of the casing looks like it's drying out, lightly mist it. Don't give it too much water because this increases the risk of waterlogging and contamination.

Fruiting and harvesting

Once the mushrooms have reached their appropriate size, you can start harvesting individual ones. Pick them when they seem like they have reached their optimal growth. Harvest them as quickly as you can because the longer you wait, the greater is the risk of them being feasted on by other critters.

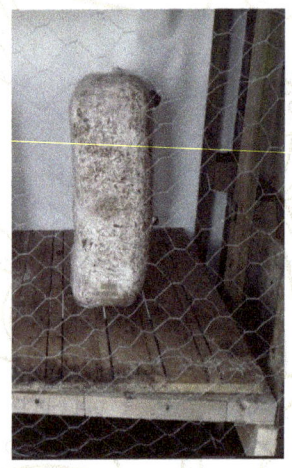

Ourdoor Environment

Outdoor Bed

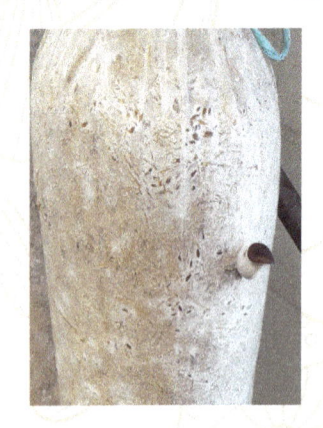

Pinning

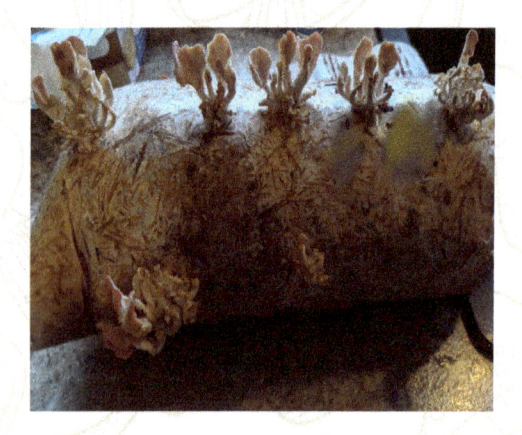

Fruiting

5. What and How to Grow

Now, let's get to the part that you were eagerly waiting for, to start growing mushrooms! It's been repeatedly mentioned that the techniques used for cultivation, including the choice of substrate and environmental factors, vary from one species of mushroom to another. Learning about the ideal growing requirements of different types of mushrooms will ensure you get a bountiful harvest! Here are the most common types of mushrooms you can start growing and their needs and requirements.

NOTE: According to the type of mushrooms you want to grow, the techniques used will also vary. Refer to the information given in the previous chapter and follow those instructions associated with the preferred growing technique.

Oyster Mushrooms

Whether you want to cultivate mushrooms at home or grow them commercially, all varieties of oyster mushrooms are a good choice. King oyster, pink oyster, pearl oyster, blue oyster, golden oyster, and phoenix oyster are different types of these mushrooms.

Depending on the variety, their size also varies. They can range from 2-10-inches.

Oyster mushrooms are saprophytic fungi that prefer subtropical and temperate forests. They usually grow on decomposing logs. The mycelium of these mushrooms belongs to the few known carnivorous fungi. The mycelium can kill and digest nematodes such as roundworms and bacteria to obtain the nitrogen required for its growth. The color of these mushrooms also depends on their variety. They can be dark grey and brown or pink, and even yellow. They have broad fan-like caps with curled edges that become waiver and lobed upon reaching full maturity. The white gills are found under the cap.

These mushrooms have a firm, white, and meaty texture. Their bittersweet aroma is quite similar to that of anise. They have a soft and slightly chewy texture with a mild nutty flavor. These mushrooms can be used as a substitute for seafood in vegan and vegetarian cooking because of their flavor and texture.

These tasty mushrooms contain a variety of nutrients such as potassium, B-complex vitamins, vitamin C, amino acids, magnesium, folic acid, and pantothenic acid. As with other mushrooms, they are also rich in vitamin D, fiber, protein, selenium, and phosphorus, calcium, and niacin.

They are believed to have immune system boosting properties, are an ideal cholesterol-free meat replacement, have anti-inflammatory properties, and prevent the buildup of plaque in the cardiovascular system.

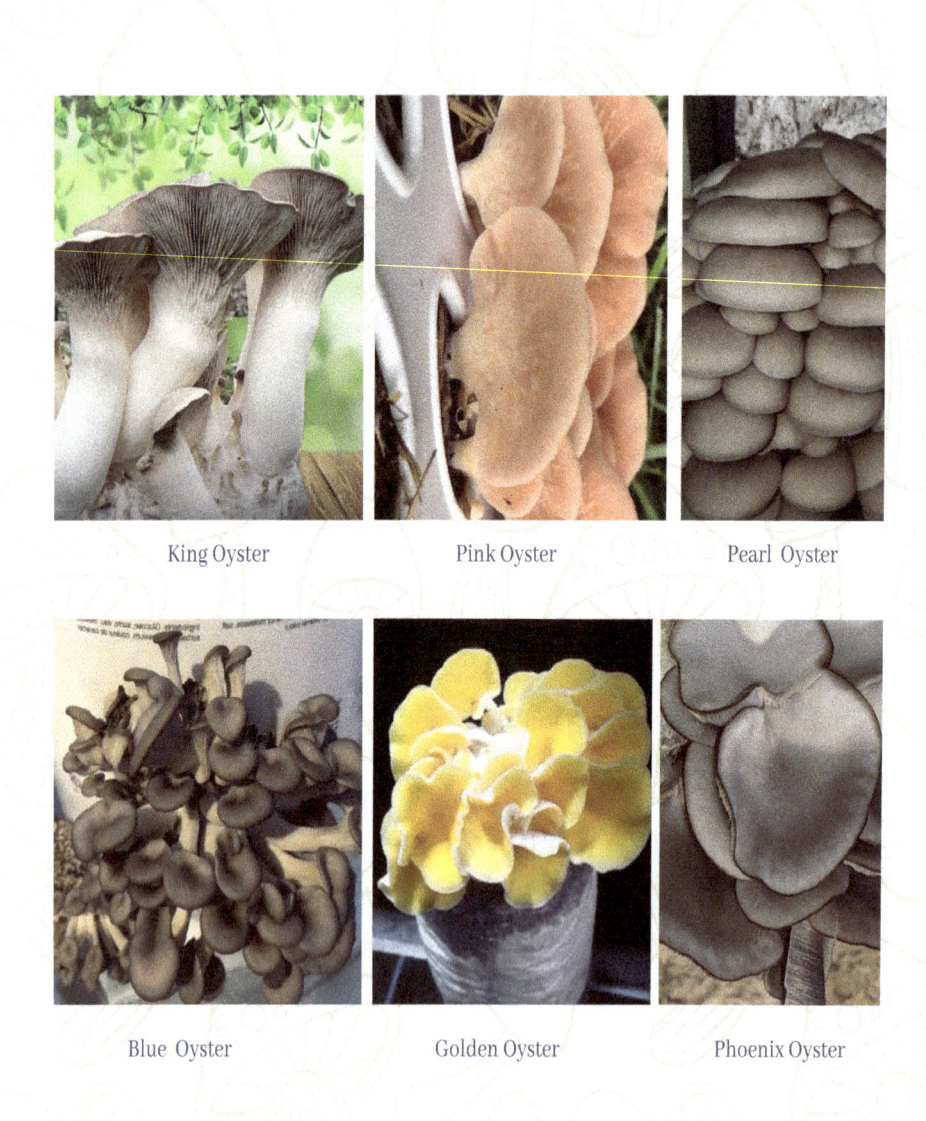

King Oyster

Pink Oyster

Pearl Oyster

Blue Oyster

Golden Oyster

Phoenix Oyster

Growing Oyster Mushrooms at Home

Oyster mushrooms are commonly found in temperate and subtropical forests, with the Pacific Northwest being a sole exception. They feed on decomposing trees, especially aspen and beech trees and other deciduous varieties. Growing these mushrooms is fairly straightforward.

You have different options available to make the mushroom spawn at home. For example, you can use wild bird seed, sawdust, and grains such as millets. There are also various substrates to choose from, but sawdust, coffee grounds, and straw are the most commonly used options.

The 5-gallon bucket method, log grow, spawn to the substrate, and PF Tek are the cultivation techniques you can use. These mushrooms can be grown both outdoors and indoors, depending on the method you are using.

A shotgun fruiting chamber works for the PF Tek method, while a grow bag or the 5-gallon bucket method is ideal for growing the mushrooms from spawn to substrate.

The ideal time to harvest them is as soon as their caps start turning upward or flatten out. The mushroom starts dropping spores if you wait for too long, and their taste deteriorates. Grab the mushroom at its base and twist and tug it gently to harvest. Alternatively, use a sharp knife to cut the mushroom as close to the base as you possibly can. If you don't want to consume these mushrooms immediately, you can dry them and store.

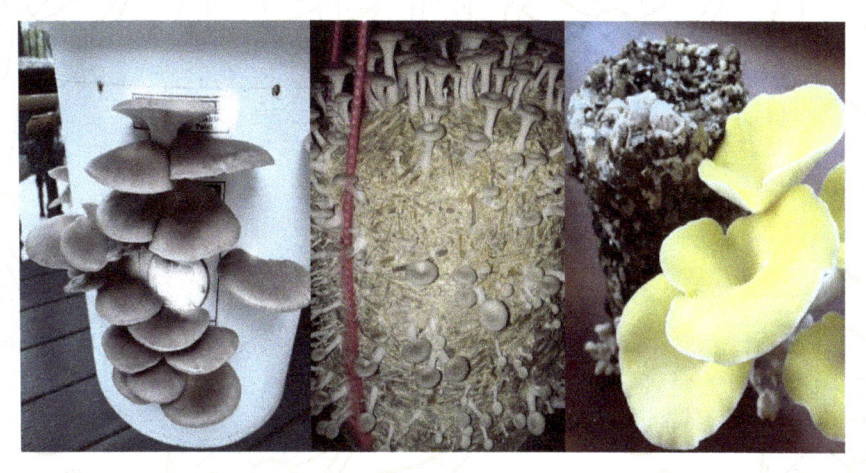

5-gallon bucket- Blue Osyter   Grow Bag Method- Grey Oyster   PF Tek - Golden Oyster

Lion's Mane

It is a unique species of mushrooms. It has an almost hair-like appearance when it's fully mature and resembles a lion's mane, and thus its name. The fruits can be anywhere between 4-10 inches big when they are fully ripe. It is one of the most common saprophytic mushrooms in North America, including Canada and the United States.

The soft and slender spines produced by this mushroom give it a mane-like appearance. These spines release their spores. They are bright white, to begin with, and turn a pale yellowish-brown as the mushroom matures. These mushrooms are not unique to look at but taste incredibly delicious as well. They are extremely tender and have a slightly chewy consistency with a mild and sweet flavor. These mushrooms are quite similar in flavor and texture to scallops, lobster, and crab. So, they are a brilliant substitute for seafood.

These mushrooms are believed to promote the growth of brain cells while alleviating symptoms of anxiety and depression. In addition, their anti-inflammatory properties are also associated with a reduced risk of heart diseases and stomach ulcers. Apart from it, they are rich in antioxidants and can assist in weight loss.

Growing Lion's Mane at Home

Depending on the cultivation technique you want to use, the substrate will also vary. While using the PF Tek method, the ideal substrate combines vermiculite and brown rice flour. For other methods, you can use hardwood chips as well. These mushrooms usually grow on dying and decaying hardwood trees and are commonly found throughout Northern America. The fruits start appearing during fall. Again, depending on the cultivation technique you are using, growing these mushrooms can be incredibly easy or even slightly tricky.

Different varieties of grain make the ideal spawn for a lion's mane. The best-suited grain for this species is rye. However, whenever you are growing the spawn, its mycelium looks quite wispy and thin. So, it will take a while before you can tell whether the spawn is fully colonized or not.

Don't forget to check the spawn in bags or jars to ensure optimal colonization. Adding hardwood sawdust to the spawn is ideal for this specific species. The sawdust can also be supplemented with 10-20% of wheat bran.

The possible growing techniques include log growth, grain or sawdust, and PF Tek. These mushrooms can be grown both indoors and outdoors, depending on climatic factors. Depending on the technique you decide to use, the fruiting chamber will also vary. If you are opting for PF Tek, a shotgun fruiting chamber does the trick. A grow bag works well when you are spawning the mushrooms from grain to sawdust. If you are growing it outdoors, provided the suitable climatic conditions, the log grow technique is ideal.

To harvest the fruit, cut the mushroom as close to its base as you possibly can using a sharp knife and avoid tugging on them. Ensure that you don't damage their spines while harvesting. You can store these fruits in the fridge for later.

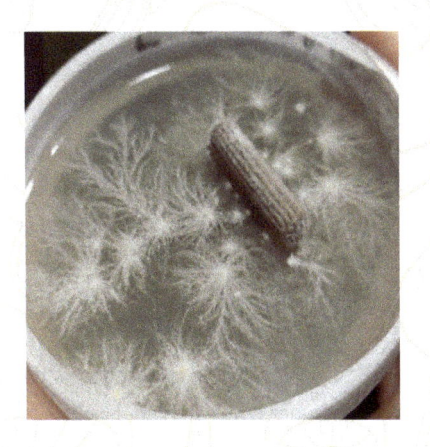

Inoculation of Lion's Mane in an Agar Dish

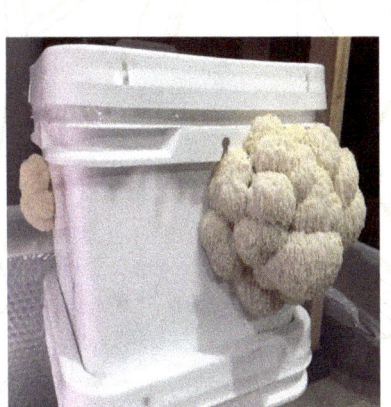

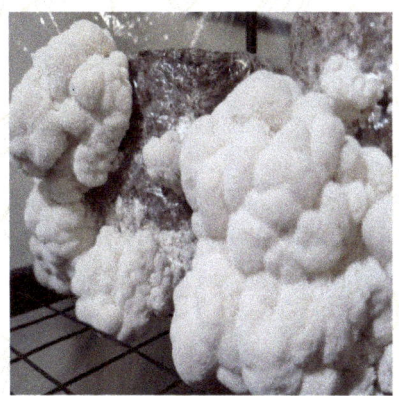

Lion's Mane in Grow Bag

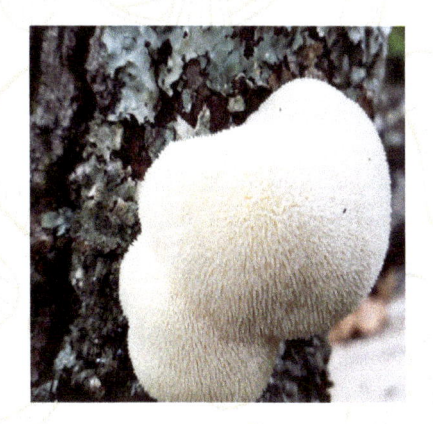

Lion's Mane in 5 Gallon Bucket

Lion's Mane on Maple Log

Reishi

Unlike the other mushrooms discussed in this section, the reishi mushrooms fall into the category of medicinal mushrooms instead of edible ones. A distinguishing factor of this specific species is they don't have any gills. The tiny pores present under the cap release its spores.

It has a kidney-shaped cap that's reddish-brown colored with a varnished appearance. When fully mature, they resemble a fan-like structure. The pores are generally white to start with and slowly turn brown as the mushroom ages. Different varieties of these mushrooms are commonly found in North America and Asia. They can be saprotrophic and even parasitic. That means, in the wild, these mushrooms are found on trees that are not only living but dead as well.

As mentioned, these mushrooms are generally consumed for various health and medicinal benefits they offer. It has a soft, almost cork-like texture. These mushrooms have been used in traditional medicine across most of eastern Asia for hundreds of years now. Some historical records of these mushrooms being used in China go back to 104 BCE. Some also believe these mushrooms not only offer medicinal healing but spiritual healing as well.

These mushrooms are believed to strengthen immune functioning by tackling inflammation. Some claim it fights different types of cancer by increasing the activity of white blood cells. Regular consumption of these mushrooms and their extracts can improve the overall quality of one's life while elevating symptoms of depression and anxiety. These mushrooms are also believed to regulate blood sugar levels while improving cardiovascular health.

Growing Reishi at Home

Reishi Mushrooms are native to the regions of Asia and North America but they grow from the stumps of deciduous trees. Maple is their preferred wood. These mushrooms can be grown both indoors and outdoors. That said, growing them is moderately difficult. The growing techniques you can use are PF Tek, 5-gallon bucket method and log grow technique. The difficulty level of growing this mushroom is directly proportional to the cultivation technique you decide to grow. The best food source for the mushroom spawn is sawdust in this case. Sawdust, hardwood log, or hardwood chips are the ideal substrates for growing reishi mushrooms.

You can also combine any of these woods gypsum and brand to get a good spawn as well.

Depending on the climatic factors, these mushrooms can be grown both outdoors and indoors. While using the PF Tek method, you will need a shotgun fruiting chamber. When it comes to any of the spawn to substrate methods, you can use grow bags, a 5-gallon bucket, or a monotub as the fruiting chamber.

Harvesting these mushrooms is incredibly simple. You need to use a gentle twist and tug method. Twist the mushrooms from their base and try not to damage them while doing this. Alternatively, you can cut them with a sharp knife. Once these mushrooms are dried, you can store them for prolonged periods. If you want to use them immediately or within a short period, store them in the fridge.

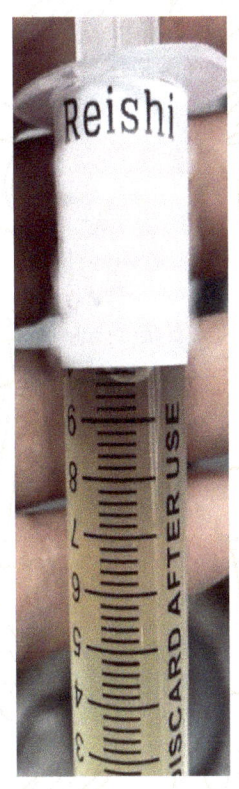

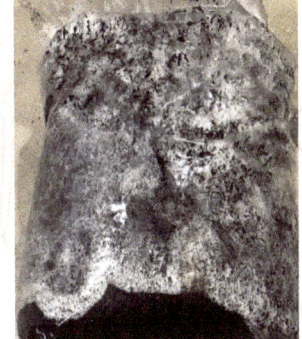

Colonization

Fruiting

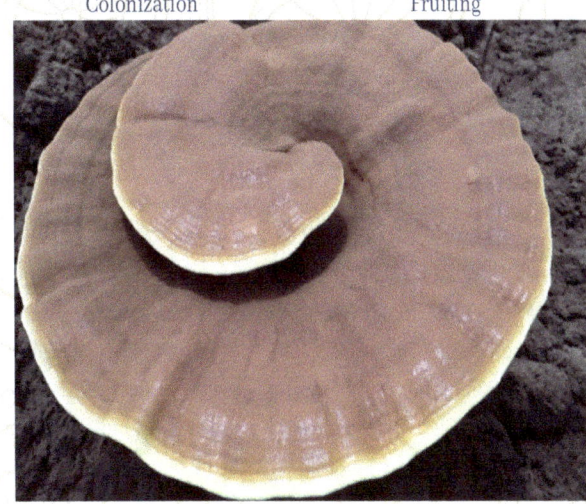

Strain of Reishi

Reishi Mushroom

Wine Cap

The caps of this medium to large-sized mushrooms are reddish burgundy when young. This is where the mushrooms get their name. They typically have 2–5-inch white caps with long and thick stems. As the mushrooms mature, the cap turns yellowish-brown and starts drying up. The ideal time to pick these mushrooms is when they are relatively young to ensure the best flavor.

These mushrooms are ideal for growing outdoors. If you have a vegetable garden outside, grow these mushrooms along with them. They belong to the agaric family of Stropharia. Wine caps are one of the few edible mushrooms that belong to this genus. They are saprophytic fungi that grow on decomposing wood, including wood chips. They are also known as Godzilla mushrooms, garden giants, and king Stropharia. Once the mushrooms are fully mature, they can weigh up to 5 lbs. These mushrooms have a firm and nice white stem and flesh that's usually cooked and consumed. They have a crisp texture with an almost nutty and earthy flavor. Some believe their flavor profile includes hints of red wine and potatoes.

These mushrooms have different health benefits and medicinal properties. They are commonly used as a low-calorie meat substitute because of their flavor and texture. They are low in calories, have almost no cholesterol or any unhealthy fats. They are an excellent source of proteins. These mushrooms are believed to reduce and regulate blood sugar and cholesterol levels.

Growing Wine Cap at Home

The ideal environment for growing them is outdoors. That said, you can also grow them indoors, but the results will not be as good as the ones derived from those grown outdoors. These mushrooms are native to Europe, North America, New Zealand, and Australia.

Growing these mushrooms is moderately easy. The possible growing techniques you can use are an outdoor mushroom bed or any other method where you grow from spawn to substrate. The ideal spawn for wine caps is sawdust, and their ideal substrates include compost, hardwood chips, and sawdust. Since you will be growing these mushrooms outdoors, you don't need any specific fruiting chambers associated with indoor growth.

To harvest these mushrooms, simply pinch them at the base and gently twist and pull. Alternatively, they can be cut with a sharp knife as well. When stored in the fridge, they can last for up to a week.

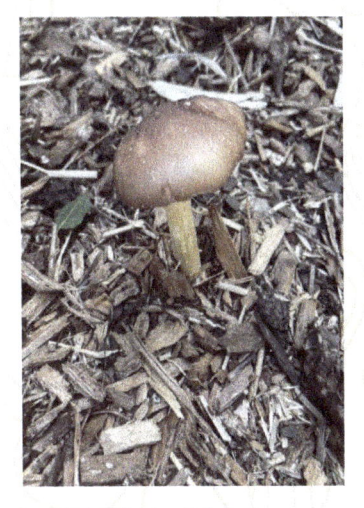

Saw Dust as Substrate   Wine Cap Harvesting

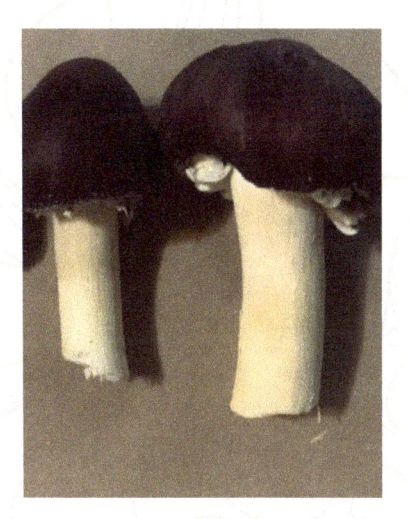

Enokitake

Enokitake mushrooms are commonly known as enoki. Depending on where and how they are grown, the appearance of Enokitake mushrooms differs. The color and length of these mushrooms are based on environmental factors.

For instance, they are thin with long stems and are bright white when they are grown in a carbon dioxide-rich environment devoid of light. On the other hand, if they are exposed to sufficient light, they develop a golden-brown tinge. The cultivated varieties of these mushrooms are quite different from the ones found in the wild. The saprotrophic wild Enokitake usually grows on tree stumps, is thick and short, and dark brown colored. Depending on whether you decide to cultivate these species with light exposure or not, you will end up with golden or white Enokitake, respectively. If you want a tightly packed cluster of small capped and long and thin fruits, a carbon dioxide-rich environment is important. These tender and crisp mushrooms have a mild peppery flavor. They are commonly used in East Asian cuisine. These mushrooms are not only a pretty sight but are incredibly tasty and nutritious as well.

They are filled with dietary fiber, healthy protein, essential minerals, and vitamins, along with a variety of antioxidants. These mushrooms are believed to fight inflammation, boost immune functioning, and improve cardiovascular health.

Growing Enokitake at Home

In the wild, these mushrooms are commonly found on dead conifer trees and Chinese hackberry trees. Depending on how you decide to grow them, the yield and appearance vary. When compared to other mushrooms, these are relatively trickier to grow. Aged hardwood sawdust or paper products along with certain types of seeds and grains are the best media for spawning these mushrooms.

Compost, sawdust, wood chips, and straw are the best substrates for enoki mushrooms.

Compost, sawdust, wood chips, and straw are the best substrates for enoki mushrooms.

Growing these mushrooms outdoors is not the best idea. Even if you decide to grow them outdoors, the container or enclosure in which you are growing them needs to be shielded from direct sunlight. To grow typical Enokitake mushrooms, you need a CO_2-rich environment with as little light as possible. The ideal fruiting temperature for these mushrooms is between 40 and 60°F. You can grow them in plastic or glass jars, grow bags, and monotub as well. To harvest, simply pull a cluster. You can also store them in the fridge for later consumption.

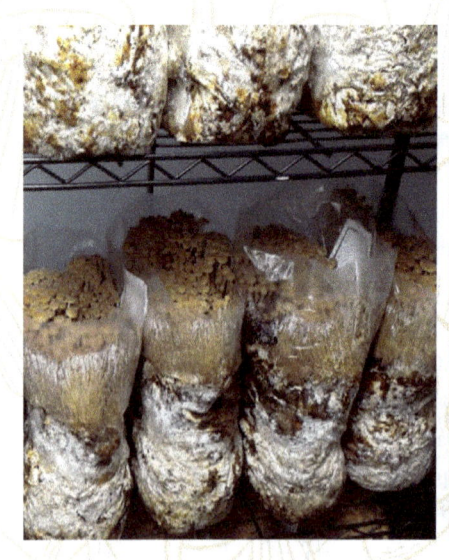

Colonization in Substrate

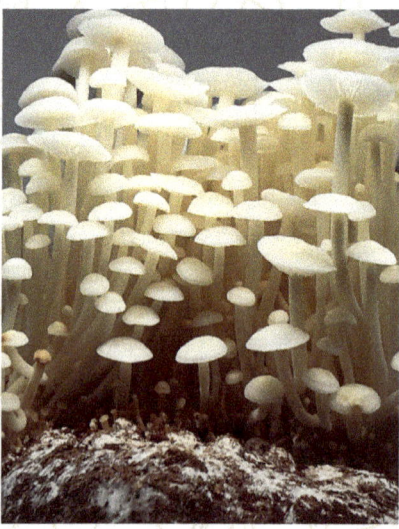

Enoki Fruiting

Black Poplar

Black poplar mushrooms are also known as velvet pioppini. These small to medium-sized mushrooms are characterized by pretty long stems and caps anywhere between 1 and 4-inches wide.

Depending on their level of maturity and the area where they are grown, the caps range from light to dark brown. The dark gills present under the caps release the mushroom spores. These mushrooms usually grow on stumps of different trees worldwide, including the black poplar and hence their name.

These mushrooms are not only edible but have been a part of traditional Chinese medicine for ages. The texture and taste of these mushrooms are quite similar to asparagus. They are crunchy and savory with a slightly peppery, earthy, sweet, and nutty flavor profile. Their flavor and texture make an excellent addition to stews, pasta, and soups.

These mushrooms are rich in various minerals, vitamins, and amino acids without harmful calories or cholesterol. Some common nutrients include B-complex vitamins, copper, pantothenic acid, potassium, folate, and niacin. In traditional Chinese medicine, these mushrooms are used to cure nausea, fever, and headaches. They are also believed to have anti-inflammatory and anti-fungal properties.

Growing Black Poplar at Home

These mushrooms are found around chestnut, poplar, elm, willow, and maple trees in the wild. Depending on the cultivation technique you are using, growing them ranges from relatively easy to moderately tricky. The ideal spawn includes grain, seeds, and sawdust, while the best substrates are grains, hardwood logs, sawdust, and wood chips. Some possible growing techniques you can use are log grows, PF Tek, and any method where you need to grow both the spawn and the substrate. Using the PF Tek method, you will need a shotgun fruiting chamber and monotub or grow bag for any spawn to substrate methods.

Grab the mushroom at its base and use a gentle twist and pull to harvest them. Always cut these mushrooms as close to their base as you can. These mushrooms can be dried and stored for prolonged periods or consumed immediately.

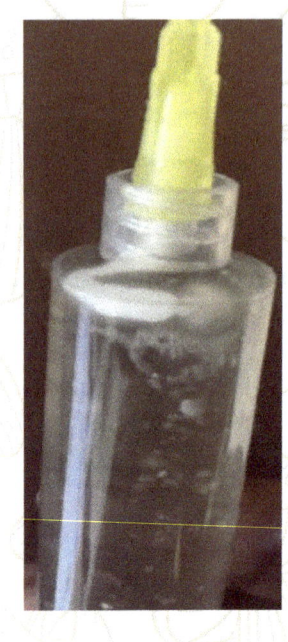

Black Poplar Culture

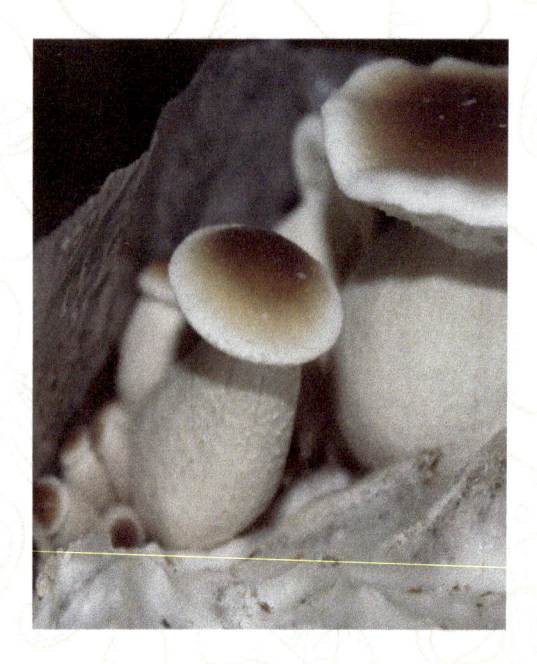

Black Poplar Fruiting

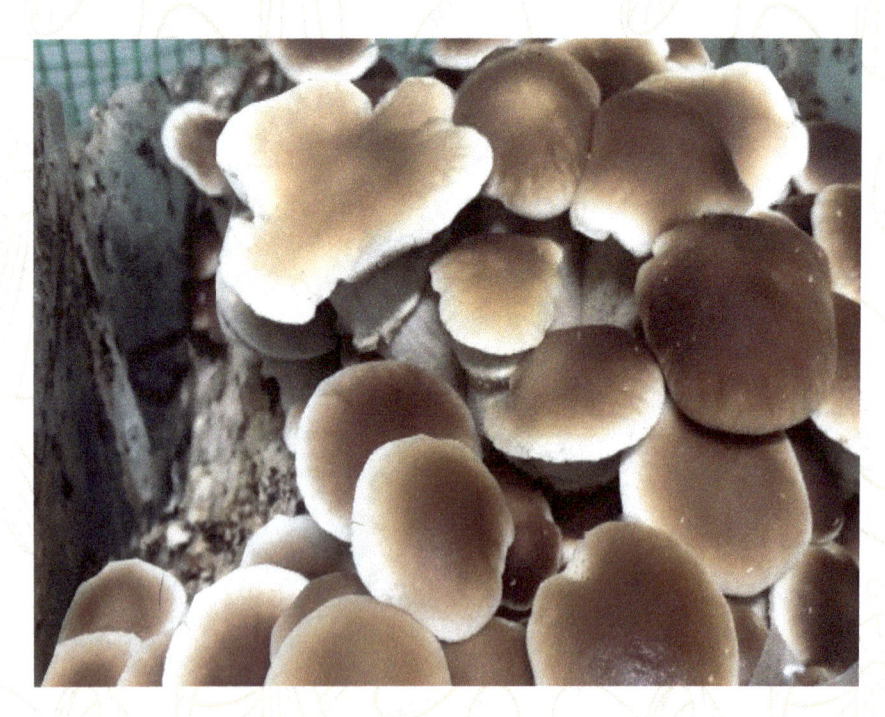

Black Poplar - Ready to Harvest

Shiitake

One of the most popular mushrooms across the globe is the shiitake. You can easily purchase them from any local grocery store but growing them at home is an incredibly rewarding and enjoyable process.

These small to medium-sized mushrooms have caps that can be anywhere between 4-8 inches wide. Shiitake mushrooms are saprophytic fungi commonly found in clusters along with those hardwood trees. They are predominantly native to East Asia, especially China and Japan. These mushrooms are not only delicious but are used for medicinal reasons as well.

These mushrooms have a slightly spongy and chewy texture with cream-colored flesh inside the cap. The stem can be ivory to brown colored. Both the stem and the cap of these mushrooms have a fibrous texture. It has a pleasant savory, earthy, umami, and smoky flavor. They can be cooked in different ways ranging from grilling to frying and baking and even boiling. These mushrooms are not only used in Asian cooking but can be added to pretty much any recipe that calls for earthy textures.

These delicious fungi are believed to reduce blocks in the cardiovascular system, improve heart health, and reduce harmful fats in the body. They also have antimicrobial properties. Apart from this, these mushrooms have vitamins and nutrients important for improving your skin's health, are rich in B-complex vitamins that improve your energy levels and cognition as well.

Growing Shiitake at Home

The yields produced by the mushrooms and the difficulty involved in growing them vary according to the cultivation technique used. As mentioned, they are native to regions of South East and Eastern Asia. They thrive in warm and moist climatic conditions. In the wild, they are usually found on dead and decaying hardwood trees such as mulberry, chestnut, maple, ironwood, and poplar.

These mushrooms can be grown both indoors and outdoors. The log method, PF Tek, and spawn to substrate methods are ideal for shiitake mushrooms. The ideal spawn and substrate you can use are sawdust or grain and hardwood chips, hardwood logs, and hardwood sawdust respectively. While using PF Tek, you will need a shotgun fruiting chamber. Whereas you can use grow bags for any spawn to substrate grow. To harvest them, simply grab the fruit at its base and pull it. You can also cut them with a sharp knife. These mushrooms are ideal for long-term storage once you dry them. Dry shiitake are commonly used in Asian cuisine.

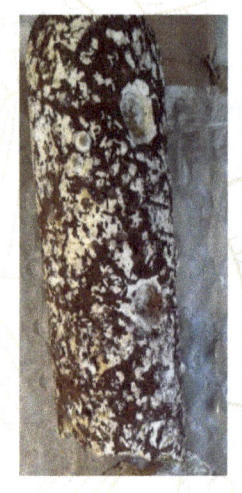

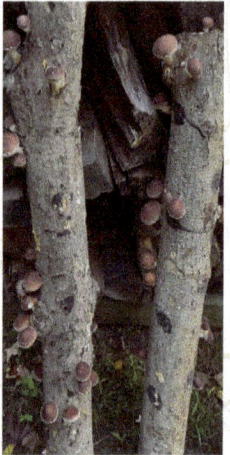

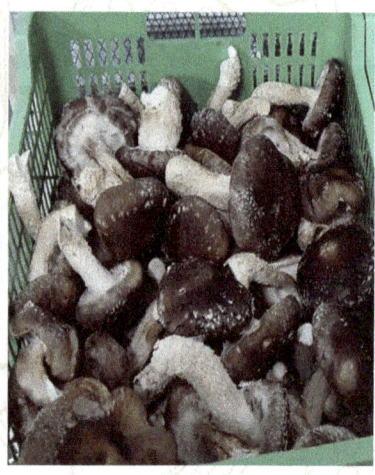

Shiitake Logs   Shiitake Flush

Maitake

Maitake mushrooms are also known as hen of the woods. In Japanese, maitake means dancing mushrooms.

These mushrooms always grow in clusters. An average cluster can weigh anywhere between 3-5 lbs. While they grow into bigger and heavier clusters in the wild. The fruiting body of these mushrooms that's visible above ground has a feathered and frilly appearance. The color of these mushroom caps varies from white to brown, depending on their level of sun exposure. The caps are wavy, smooth, and velvety to touch. The pores are present under the mushroom caps responsible for releasing the spores.

These mushrooms are not only edible but are grown for their medicinal properties as well. As a result, they are highly regarded in Japan and often grow in wild areas protected. These saprophytic fungi are commonly found on stumps of old oaks and other trees across Siberia, the eastern United States, and Japan. They usually fruit during late summer and early fall.

Maitake mushrooms are quite succulent with a slightly chewy texture when cooked. Their flavor profile has hints of earthy, spicy, and woody notes. They can be added to soups and salads when consumed fresh. Alternatively, their flavor and texture make them well suited for various cooking methods such as grilling, sautéing, frying, roasting, and even baking.

These mushrooms are extremely low in calories and have plenty of dietary fiber and protein in them. For instance, 100 grams of these mushrooms only has about 30 calories. They are rich in various essential vitamins and minerals such as vitamin D, pantothenic acid, riboflavin, folates, niacin, potassium, calcium, sodium, magnesium, manganese, phosphorus, selenium, zinc, copper, and iron. Maitake is believed to have cancer-fighting properties, tackle oxidation, regulate inflammation, strengthen immune functioning, and help regulate blood sugar levels.

Growing Maitake at Home

Growing these mushrooms is pretty tricky because the mycelium needs a specific temperature of 50-60°F. However, till you maintain the right temperature, you can grow them at home. Log grow, monotub, and grow bags can be used for these mushrooms. The ideal spawn and substrates are sawdust and grain, hardwood logs, woodchips, and sawdust. These mushrooms can be grown both indoors and outdoors, but the color of the cap varies according to their level of sun exposure.

Once these mushrooms sport their trademark frilly and feathered caps, they are ready for harvest. As with other mushrooms, the younger they are, the better they taste. These mushrooms can be frozen if you are looking for a long-term storage option

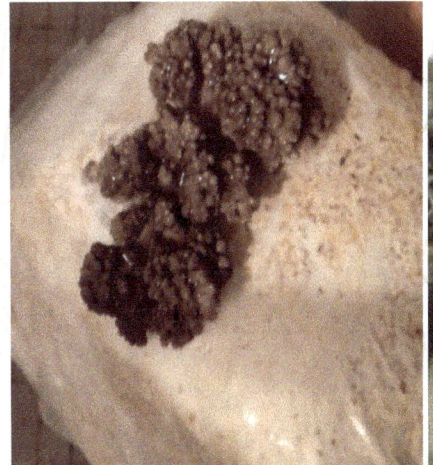

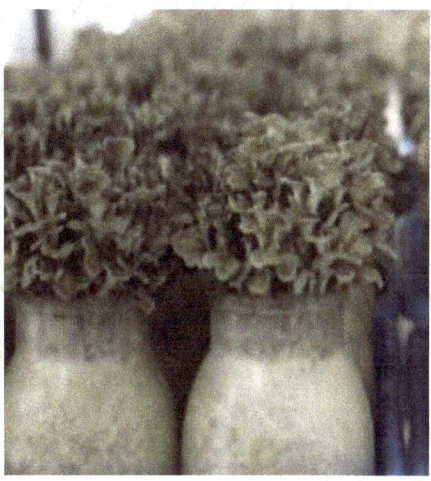

Maitake Fruiting

Maitake Farming

Luminescent Panellus

These mushrooms are neither edible nor have any medicinal properties. That said, they are grown for aesthetic appeal and are purely meant for decorative purposes. They have a bitter taste that is quite off-putting for most and therefore they are not commonly consumed.

Their bioluminescence makes these mushrooms unique. They usually appear in dense clusters on the logs and stumps of deciduous trees across the globe. Their fan-like and kidney-shaped caps can be up to 1.2-inches wide. They can be found in a variety of colors ranging from orange to yellow and even brown.

The bioluminescence is usually seen around the gills and the area where the cap and the stem are made. Its mycelium might also exhibit this property. The visible bioluminescence of these mushrooms is associated with the presence of a single dominant allele. Add these mushrooms to your house if you are interested in removing harmful pollutants and toxins from the immediate environment.

Growing Luminescent Panellus at Home

These mushrooms are found across the globe including regions of New Zealand, Europe, Japan, China, Australia, and even North America. They are commonly found on hardwood trees such as American hornbeam, pecan, birch, hickory, oak, and maple.
They are moderately easy to grow. The ideal growing techniques include log grow and spawn to substrate methods. The usually used spawn and substrates for these mushrooms include sawdust or grain and wood chips, agar, sawdust, and grain respectively. They can be grown both outdoors and indoors depending on the usual climatic conditions. As long as a moist environment is maintained, they will thrive.

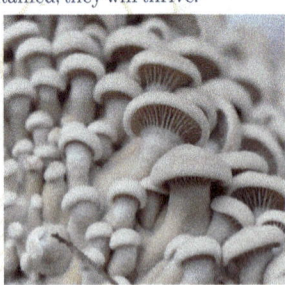

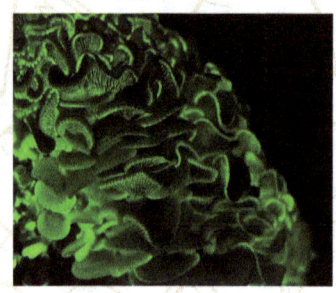

Fruiting   Glowing in Dark

6. Dealing With Common Problems

Growing mushrooms at home are not as complicated as believed. That said, there will be some obstacles or hurdles you will face along the way. Here are some common problems most beginners face while growing mushrooms. Learning to avoid them will help improve the overall yield and ensure your efforts don't go to waste.

Dealing With Contaminants

There are different reasons why mushrooms can be riddled with contaminants. The most obvious and common reason is poor sterilizing techniques. Whenever you are inoculating the substrate, ensure you use a glove box. It would help if you also used the pressure cooker to sterilize the equipment used for inoculation. Apart from this, ensure that you are wearing gloves while using the glove box. These gloves should be rubbed with 70% isopropyl alcohol before use to ensure they are perfectly sterile.

Apart from this, regularly clean the glove box and the work area. The workspace should be cleaned using a solution of bleach and water. The solution should be made of 10% bleach and 90% water. You can also use 70% Isopropyl alcohol solution or rubbing liquid as well.

Using a combination of both these techniques is a brilliant idea. Anything that you place in the glove box should also be wiped down with rubbing alcohol before placing it in the fruiting chamber or glove box. Another common source of contamination can be from the syringes used for inoculation. It is one of the reasons why the syringes should be sterilized before use. Also, you can purchase one-time-use syringes and dispose of them after every grow.

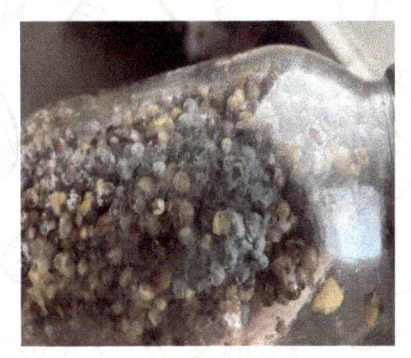

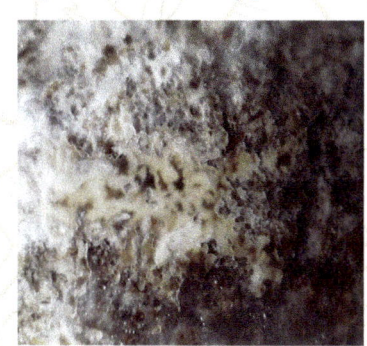

Contamination Types

Another issue that you cannot overlook is the grain used. Some strains of bacteria are heat resistant in their dormant phase. As a result, they manage to survive the temperature they are subjected to during the pressure-cooking process. The best way to ensure no traces of pesky pathogens is to soak the grain for 24-hours before sterilization. When you do this, any pathogens present in it, especially bacteria, will sprout. Once they have sprouted, the pressure-cooking process will kill them.

Even after following the suggestions mentioned, the culprit could be the growing environment if you still notice any mold. Before you select a growing area, check for mold. Check the walls, area under the sink, and all other likely places where moisture can creep in. If there is mold in the room, the chances of their spores contaminating the culture also increase.

The risk of bacterial contamination increases if too much water is added to the substrate. The grains or wood substrates you decide to use should be damp but not to the extent that they are dripping wet. Excess water in the substrate is the most common cause of bacterial contamination. If you are using grains for the substrate, ensure you don't cook them to the extent they start cracking or pop open. This increases the risk of bacterial contamination.

The temperature is one of the most important factors that you cannot overlook while growing mushrooms at home. If the environment is quite warm or you are using a heat incubation chamber, the mycelium proliferates. That said, it also makes it easier for a variety of undesirable molds to grow. Once the mycelium has matured, it is resistant to contaminants. Unfortunately, a warm environment causes the mold to grow quickly. If the mold grows more rapidly than the mycelium takes for maturation, it increases the risk of contamination.

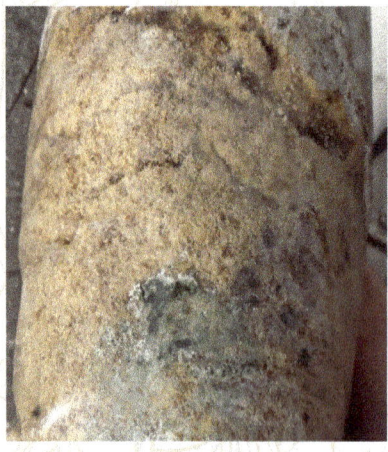

Green Mold   Black Mold

Substrate isn't Colonized

Even after doing everything right, there can be instances where nothing grows. Even after waiting for weeks, if the substrate is blank or hasn't colonized, you might unknowingly be making the mistakes discussed below.

The first factor you should consider is the temperature. Check the temperature you are colonizing. The mycelium cannot survive if it is either too hot or cold. That said, the ideal temperature requirement varies from one type of mushroom to another. Shift the substrate to another room or find a new spot to determine if the temperature is the culprit.

Apart from temperature, air circulation is another major factor at play. During the colonization phase, the substrate does not need any fresh air. However, the mycelium needs air to grow and develop. The grow bags or the jars you are using should have some provision for air circulation.

Another reason why the substrate isn't colonized could be because it is too dry. Remember, the fungus cannot grow if there is no moisture. If the substrate is too wet, it increases the risk of bacterial contamination. On the other hand, if it is too dry, it inhibits mycelial growth. So, the substrate should be moist to field capacity. Field capacity refers to the water content present in the material after the excess water is drained.

Depending on the substrate you are using, you might need to soak or boil it for longer until it reaches its field capacity. Determining the level of moisture ideal for the substrate can be a process of trial and error.

Another factor you need to pay attention to is the light available. If the jar is directly exposed to sunlight, it kills all mycelium. However, it needs a little ambient light to grow. The jars need to be placed in complete darkness for colonization. After this, exposure to a little ambient light speeds up the colonization process.

Apart from all the factors mentioned until now, if the substrate has not yet been colonized, it's probably because you have waited too long. This factor comes into play if you are using a spore print. A spore print usually contains millions of spores.

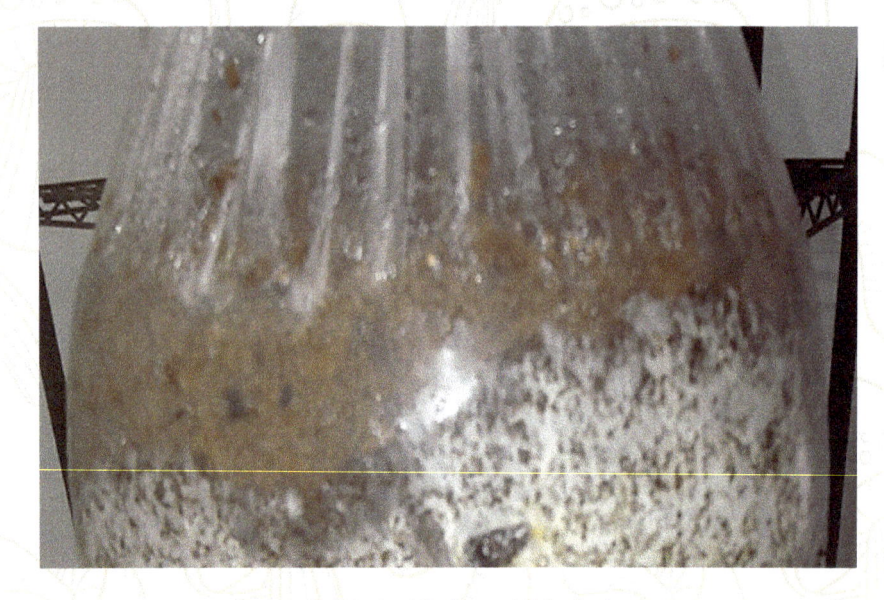

Substrate at the Top not Colonized

The genetics of these spores is not always the same. Some sprout quickly and develop mycelium, while others take a while. There will be instances when you might have to wait for months until you see any mycelial growth. If you are using spores, be patient because this process takes a while. To quicken things up, you can use a liquid culture or even agar.

The Substrate isn't Fruiting

At times, the substrate can be colonized, but it still doesn't start fruiting. If the substrate is not fruiting, significantly if you are growing indoors, environmental factors such as temperature, humidity, and light are responsible. Ensure the relative humidity is between 80- 90% for optimal fruiting conditions in the chamber. Take a spray bottle and spray down the sides of the container to maintain the desired relative humidity level.

If the temperature of the fruiting chamber is either too hot or cold, the colonized substrate doesn't bloom. Most of the common species of mushrooms do well at room temperature. That said, if the weather is extremely cold, it slows down their growth rate. Similarly, if it is too hot, it can kill the mycelium itself. If the fruiting chamber is hot, it can be due to the lighting you are using. Ensure you use a source that offers ambient lighting and doesn't produce too much heat. Suspending the light source away from the mycelium helps.

The ideal light sources include compact fluorescent or LED lights.

The indoor fruiting chamber should receive sufficient light because it is needed for pinning. You should also maintain a proper light cycle. The ambient light streaming in from a window is adequate for an indoor chamber. As long as it is not direct sunlight, it's fine. While using an artificial lighting source, ensure it is similar to the natural light cycle. It means the culture should be exposed to 12 hours of light and spend the other 12 hours in darkness. You can use a timer to ensure the culture isn't exposed to light for longer than needed.

Pinning can be delayed if there isn't sufficient fresh air. In extreme conditions, the mycelium can also completely suffocate itself to death without enough air. While using an outdoor bed, this is never an issue. This occurs only when using an indoor fruiting chamber. While using any indoor options, ensure sufficient holes in the fruiting chamber for maintaining proper airflow. If the species you are growing needs plenty of air circulation, try growing them outside instead of opting for an indoor fruiting chamber. You can also regularly fan the growing chamber to ensure that sufficient fresh air is available while excess CO_2 is expelled regularly.

If the substrate seems too dry, it is a problem that cannot be overlooked. If it looks too dry, you need to add some water to it. If using the PF Tek approach, place the pint-sized cakes in a large bowl of water and place a plate on it to keep them submerged. By soaking them for 24-hours, sufficient moisture will be reintroduced to the substrate. After this, the cakes can be reintroduced to the fruiting chamber. If you use larger cakes, place them in a bigger bucket or a plastic storage bin and repeat the process until they have sufficient moisture.

Let's consider a scenario where an outdoor growing bed is not fruiting. This can also be due to the reasons mentioned until now, such as the level of humidity, temperature, and moisture available. Ensure the substrate that is outdoors must be moist but not soaking wet. You can sprinkle it with a regular garden hose when needed. Suppose the climatic conditions in the region you reside in are arid and hot. In that case, it's better to grow the mushrooms indoors—the chances of pinning increase drastically after heavy rainfall when there is sufficient moisture in the air. Similarly, during winters, the frigid cold can result in bolting instead of fruiting.

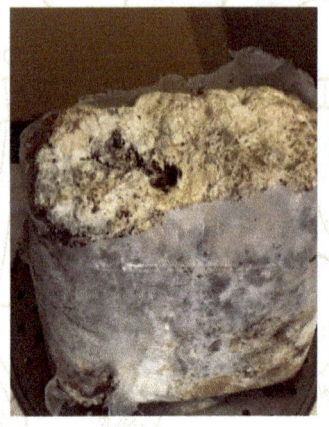

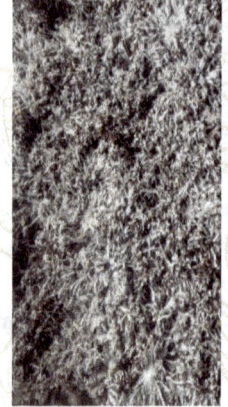

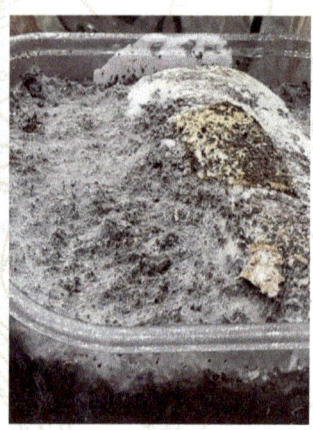

Substrate not Pinning and Fruiting

Tackling Contaminants

In the previous chapter, you were introduced to different techniques to ensure the growing equipment and the environment is sterile. When you see contaminants taking hold of the substrate or the culture, the only option is to discard the entire thing. Throwing all your efforts into a trashcan is not easy, but this is the only option once contaminated.

Therefore, make some extra effort to ensure there are no contaminants. For instance, this is the only option available when it comes to dealing with mold. Unfortunately, mold is not visible until it is too late, and by that time, it has already taken over the culture and has thoroughly contaminated and damaged it. In some cases, you can deal with the contaminant to a certain extent, such as cobwebs. Spraying a 3% hydrogen peroxide solution might help save your work, but there is no guarantee.

Mold contaminants are highly problematic because they create spores that affect the quality of the substrate and increase the chances of future contamination. This is one of the reasons why anyone growing mushrooms would throw away the substrate or the cake as soon as the first signs of mold sets in. Bacterial contaminants are relatively more forgiving than their mold counterparts. However, even this is a lost cause. As mentioned, once any contaminant sets in, it's better to discard the cake or the substrate altogether instead of trying to salvage your work. Now, let's get to fungal gnats.

They are pretty unpleasant to look at and aren't that big of a deal. Fungal gnats feed on the mycelium and mushrooms but don't ruin the entire yield. The problem with these pathogens is they leave the mycelium and mushrooms vulnerable to exposure to other sorts of contaminants.

There are different types of pests and insects that can infiltrate your mushroom garden when growing outdoors. If you aren't careful, insects, worms, birds, and other pests will feed on your mushroom garden. Once the mushrooms seem mature, harvest them immediately. Harvesting frequently also reduces the risk of other pests eating away your hard work.

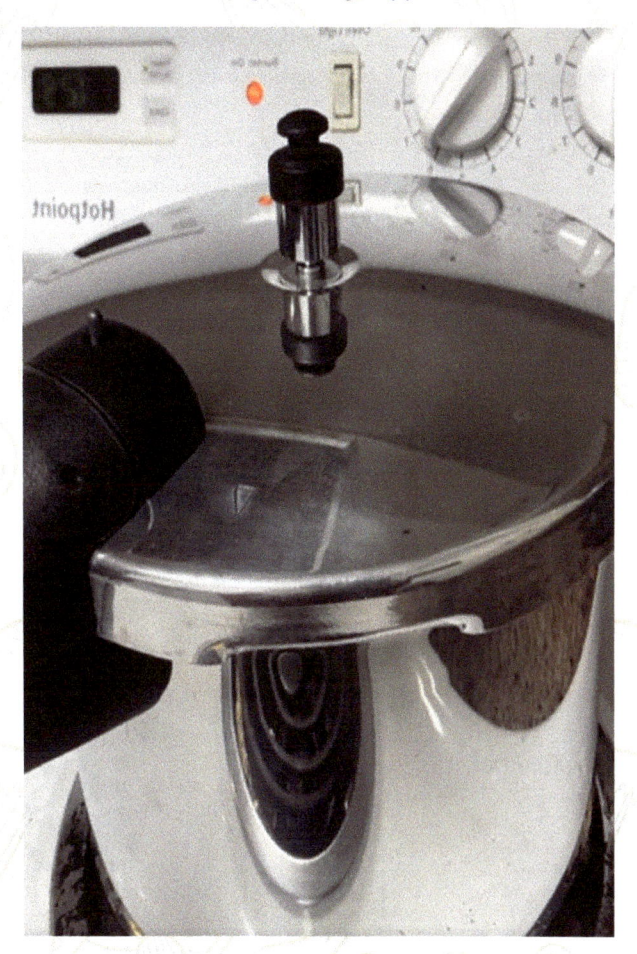

Sterilization to Control Contaminants

Small Yields

If you notice the yields are consistently small, then you will probably need to try a different technique to grow mushrooms. The yields are relatively small when you use a bottle or a jar growing technique. The same is applicable for PF Tek as well. These techniques are somewhat easier to use, but the substrate used is small. If the substrate itself is small, the yield produced will also be small. You can shift to other growing methods such as outdoor beds or monotubs to increase the yield.

Another factor responsible for small yields is the humidity level. If you are growing mushrooms using an indoor fruiting chamber such as a monotub, water droplets must be visible inside the chamber. You can ensure relative humidity levels stay ideal for mycelium growth by spraying the chamber with a little water a couple of times daily. To accurately monitor the humidity levels, you can also add a hygrometer. The relative humidity level for mushrooms to grow and thrive is 80-90%.

Depending on the species of mushrooms you are growing, their requirement for fresh air also differs. For instance, maitake and oyster mushrooms need fresh air to thrive. Therefore, chances of a good yield reduce if you try to grow such species using an indoor fruiting chamber. You can shift to a log grow or an outdoor bed to improve the yields. To improve air circulation, don't forget to add a small fan to the tank of the indoor fruiting chamber. Alternatively, simply putting a fan in the room where the fruiting chamber is placed also helps improve the airflow. This helps reduce the carbon dioxide levels and introduces fresh air to the mycelium.

The genetics of the mushrooms also matters when it comes to the yield. If you are inoculating from a spore print or syringe or using a liquid culture made from spores providing only small yields, you cannot expect a better yield. It is because the genetic traits of the spores in the print or syringe vary greatly. As mentioned, some take longer to bloom than others. Similarly, their yield also differs. Fix this situation by using a liquid or an agar culture that is created by using the clones of high-yielding mushroom varieties.

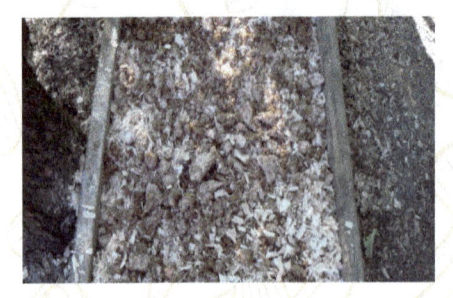

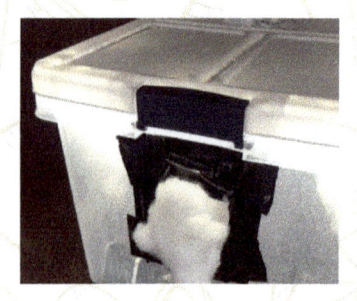

Outdoor Bed   Monotub

7. Earning Profits by Growing Mushrooms

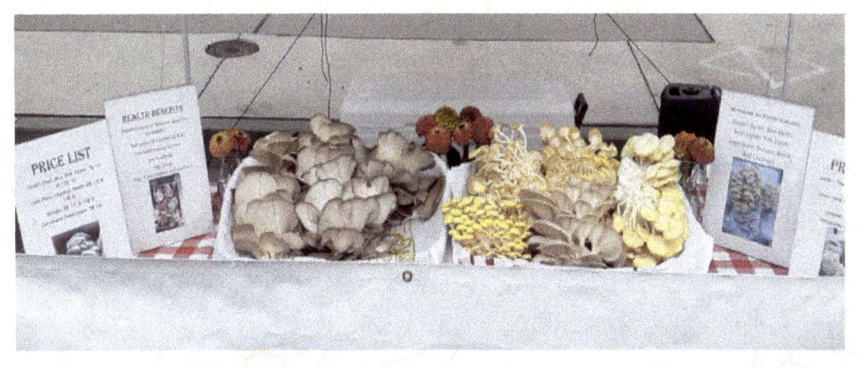

Mushroom Stall

If you have started enjoying the process of cultivating mushrooms at home and are incredibly happy with the fresh yields, consider turning it into a business. Yes, you read it right! You can start earning money by selling mushrooms grown at home. Walk into any supermarket or grocery store, and you'll see varieties of mushrooms to choose from. Well, even these stores need to get their supplies from somewhere. You can become a supplier. There are different options available when it comes to earning profits by growing mushrooms at home.

A wonderful thing about growing mushrooms at home is it was cost-effective. You don't need any massive investment. Even if the startup costs are relatively high, the process and yield pay for themselves. Before you start thinking about earning profits by starting a mushroom business, you need to have a thorough understanding of the cultivation process and techniques used. From preparing the spawn and substrate to incubation, fruiting and harvesting, these steps cannot be ignored.

There's always a demand for mushrooms in the existing market. This is one of the reasons why starting a business on your own is a wonderful idea. Most mushrooms are used as meat substitutes in vegan and vegetarian recipes. With the growing awareness of healthy plant-based diets, the popularity of mushrooms is also steadily increasing. This, coupled with all the different benefits associated with them discussed in the previous chapters, makes mushrooms incredibly nutritious.

Another wonderful thing about mushrooms is they come in different varieties. Apart from the ones discussed in the previous section, different species can be cultivated at home. You simply need to select a growing technique, perfect it, and start growing the washroom you want to sell. Yes, it is as easy as that. So come on, let's learn more about how you can make a profit by turning to mushroom cultivation.

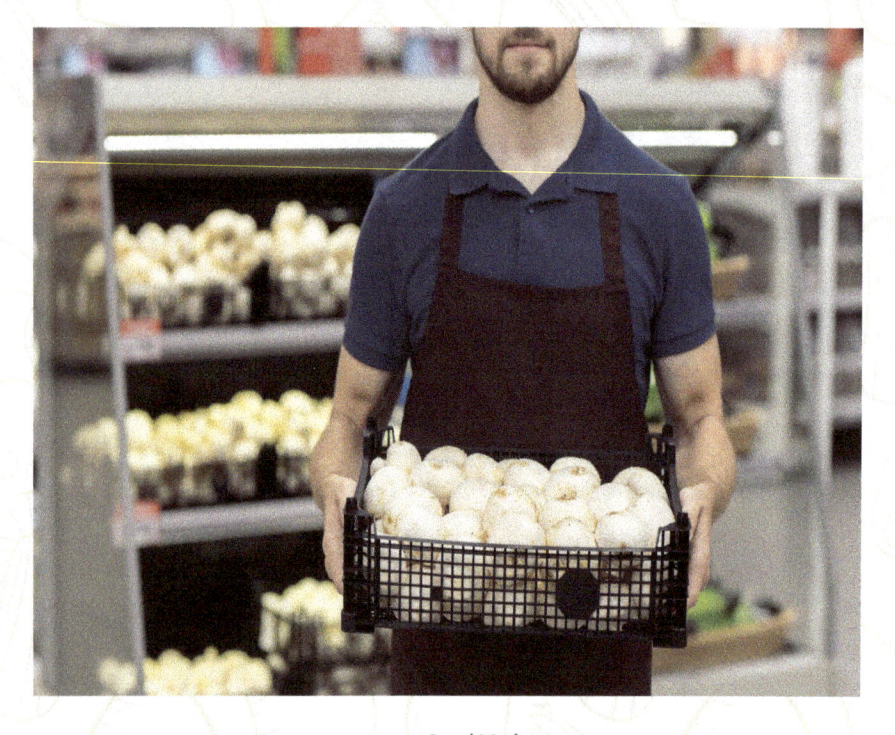

Local Market

Checking the Local Stores

If you want to start a business, you need to have a plan in place. There is no way around this. Unless you have a proper business plan, you cannot become profitable or successful. As with anything else in life, failing to plan is equivalent to planning to fail. If this is not your aim, spend some time and create a business plan. This includes the type of mushrooms you want to grow, the technique involved in the process, the time taken to grow, and how you want to distribute the said mushrooms. You should also consider a profit margin while doing this.

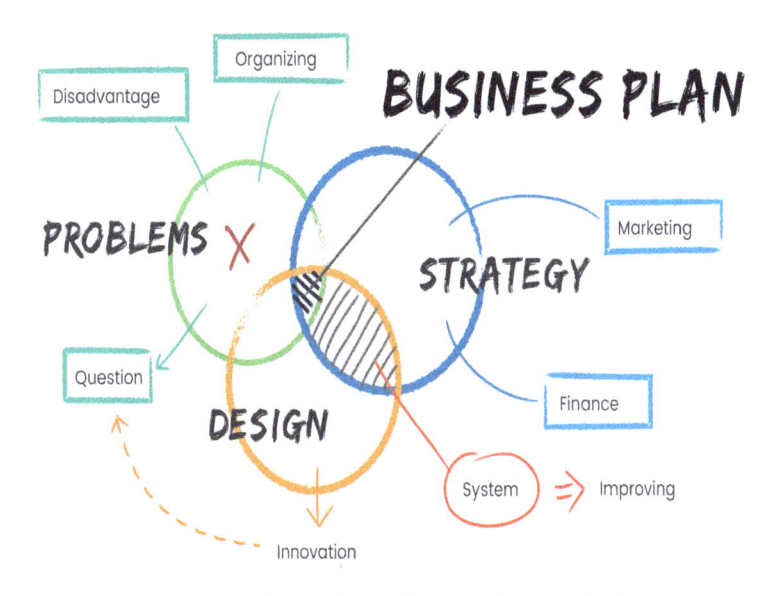

Business Plan

The simplest way to go about this process is by checking the local retail price of mushrooms. Check the prices at local supermarkets, grocery stores, and even farmer's markets. Consider all these prices and check how your competitors are pricing their products. While calculating the costs and profits involved, take into consideration the capital invested for making the spawn, substrate, and cultivation techniques. After this, you should also consider the marketing and advertising costs along with transportation.
\
Are you wondering if there is sufficient demand for mushrooms that you are growing? Some reports suggest that mushroom consumption has been increasing by about 23.5 million lbs in the United States alone. The higher the demand, the higher the selling price. This, in turn, means the greater the chance of becoming profitable.

Mushroom farming businesses have become quite trendy these days. Your business will be even more profitable when you start marketing it as an organic product. You don't need any chemicals to grow mushrooms. With the steadily increasing demand for organic produce, selling mushrooms grown at home without using any harmful chemicals will become a selling point.

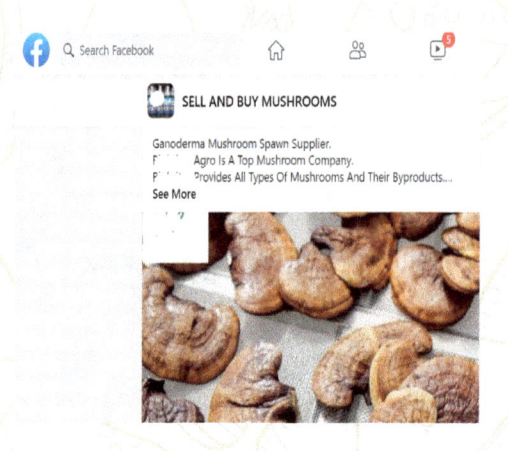

Using Social Media

It's not just about growing mushrooms; if you want to be profitable, you need to have a selling plan in place of work. The selling plan shouldn't be restricted to just whom you want to sell but should consider your marketing and trading strategies as well. You need both online and offline marketing and advertising strategies to be successful in this ultra-digitized world we live in.

From leveraging the power of social media to create a presence for your business to using newsletters and other online platforms to stay in touch with customers, there are different things you must consider.

Some Basic Concepts

Now that you have found the perfect business idea, it's time to take the next step. Starting a business is so much more than getting it registered in the state you reside in.

Business Plan

You should always start with a clear business plan. Business owners need plenty of space to grow mushrooms, especially if they want to become profitable. You can grow up to 12,000 lbs of mushrooms annually within a 500 sq ft area. That said, you need to have a proper plan in place to cater to the humidity, temperature, and lighting requirements of mushrooms you want to grow. Other upfront costs you must consider include investing in a space heater, humidifier, or dehumidifier, depending on the climatic conditions of the area you reside.

You will also need to purchase the required spores and growing medium. Depending on the technique used, the spores or spawn and substrate of the growing medium will vary.

While creating the business plan, make a list of your target market. Some examples were covered in the previous section. Consider the selling price and profit margin. Calculate the profitability while considering all the expenses mentioned until now.

You can also think about creating additional earnings from mushroom cultivation by selling DIY mushroom growing kits or conducting classes and workshops on growing mushrooms.

Legal Entity

If you want to become an entrepreneur, you need a business. Your homegrown mushroom business will not be legal until you register it. The most common business structures ideal for this venture include establishing a partnership, sole proprietorship, corporation, or even a limited liability company (LLC).

When you establish the business as an LLC or a corporation, it protects you from personal liability. However, you cannot protect your assets and wealth unless you register the business as a separate legal entity. To avoid personal liability, don't opt for sole proprietorship and partnership.

All legal entities are liable to pay their taxes. This includes local, state, and federal taxes. So, even your mushroom business is liable to pay all the applicable taxes. The taxation rules and regulations differ from one state to another. Don't forget to carefully check all the required guidelines to ensure you aren't committing a felony. Before you open the business, register it for all the applicable taxes. Hire a lawyer or a chartered accountant if you think you cannot do this on your own. It is always better to err on the side of caution!

To further protect your assets, you will need to establish a dedicated business banking account and credit account. If you start mixing your accounts with the business ones, you'll end up risking your personal finances and assets.

Apart from it, it will also get you into trouble with the law. Building business credit makes it easier to obtain the required financing options for scaling the business in the future. From obtaining higher lines of credit to better interest rates, there's a lot to gain by creating an excellent financial profile and credit for your business. You will need a dedicated business account for recording all business expenses as well. This will make it easier to determine how well your business is performing and its financial health. Apart from it, once you have all the accounts in order, it becomes easier to file taxes during the year-end.

Permits and Licenses

Not acquiring the required permits and licenses will land your business in hot water. You can also run into legal trouble. In the worst-case scenario, it might mean your business will be shut down, and you will not be allowed to operate another similar business. Since it is a business, check the local laws and regulations and obtain the required permits and licenses.

Apart from permits and licenses, ensure you create detailed contracts
whenever you are acting as a supplier for other businesses. Whether it's a local chef, restaurant, or even grocery store, ensure you have legally binding documents in place. These documents should not only specify what you will be doing, the services provided, but the costs incurred and payable along with the dispute resolution techniques. When you have these legally binding documents in place, the risk of running into any legal trouble reduces. This also becomes easier to take the required legal action when others default.

Business Insurance

Apart from licenses and permits, your business also needs insurance. Insurance ensures your business is running lawfully and safely. It protects the financial wellbeing of your business on the happening of an event covered by it. Different types of insurance policies are available, and they are created for varying businesses with varying levels of risk. If you are unsure of the specific type of insurance your business needs, you are going with general liability insurance does the trick. This is the most common type of coverage opted for by small businesses.

Defining Your Brand

It's not just about creating a business; you should also create a brand for this business. How others view your business as the brand. For instance, seeing a brightly colored or illuminated capital M probably reminds you of McDonald's while the sign of a tick mark on shoes will remind you of Nike. This is how brands work. The idea of creating a brand is to create an impression in the minds of people. This makes it easier to increase customer loyalty while creating a social standing you're your business. Another important function of creating a brand for business is it helps you stand apart from your competitors.

To create a brand, you'll need to think about promoting and market the mushroom business. There is a lot to do from interpersonal interactions, including conversations with potential clients to create online advertising and digital frameworks. If you are not comfortable doing all this, do not hesitate to ask for help and hire professionals to do this for you. It's always better to concentrate on the areas of business you are familiar and comfortable with. This ensures the right person is doing the right job. This, in turn, will improve the efficiency, effectiveness, and profitability of your business. You will also need a plan in place to retain your existing customers while attracting new ones. Whether you are introducing them to different recipes for cooking healthy dishes using mushrooms or want to start a workshop, think of what you can do to increase the business's popularity.

While creating a brand, you should also consider making a business website. The world we live in has been revolutionized by technology. These days everyone has an online presence, and your business shouldn't be any different. The simplest way to create an online presence is by creating a website. Invest time and energy to create a business website. Once again, you can hire or outsource this responsibility to professionals. The business website is the digital counterpart to your business's brick-and-mortar store. Even if you don't have a physical outlet, it is okay, but ensure you have a website.

Basic Goals of a Business

The primary goal of any business is to earn profit. This would be your goal for starting a mushroom business as well. After all, you'll need to see some results for the efforts you're making. Just come in the form of profitability. The thing about profits is it is so much more than just numbers and figures. It would help if you also considered the efforts involved in keeping the business afloat. An important aspect of running a business is maintaining the right mindset. Instead, you need to let go of any limiting beliefs and shift all your attention to what you are doing

Limiting beliefs can be paralyzing, and they will prevent you from even getting started. To avoid this:

- Start believing in your business idea.
- Don't invest more than you can lose.
- Consider your risk exposure while creating a business plan to increase the chances of success

The efforts involved in running the business cannot be overlooked. A simple way to go about doing this is by using the 80/20 rule. This rule suggests that 20% of the efforts should account for 80% of the total results produced. Once you start doing this, your profitability will automatically improve. This rule comes in handy while deciding asset allocation as well. Since resources are always finite with infinite uses, it is crucial to ensure they are put to the right use.

While starting and running your business, remember that you don't have to do everything yourself. This is not only unrealistic, but it is impossible. No one can be good at everything. If your strengths include growing mushrooms and people skills, use these two skills to your absolute advantage. Instead of wasting your time, resources, and energy doing things you cannot, concentrate on doing what you know and do it to the best of your abilities. All the other responsibilities can be delegated and outsourced. You need to manage the resources you hire or use to get things done.

8. Frequently Asked Questions

Over the years, I have been part of several Mushroom Growers communities, both offline and online. As a result, I maintain a notebook in all the discussions to jot down the main queries, issues, and suggested solutions.

Below are the 10 beginner questions and proposed answers by multiple cultivators and sellers. I hope you would appreciate the diverse solutions to the common problem and try based on your situation.

1. I am just starting out, give some beginner tips?

- Get a kit online to try it out.
- Join online and offline communities for beginners.
- Invest time on YouTube channels like FreshCap or Northspore, or others to learn about growing mushrooms.
- Figure out where to grow mushrooms in your house. Whether it would be indoor or outdoor areas? Also, watch mushroom growth in nature as often as possible!
- Have clarity on where you want to go with this, just for hobby or potential business in mind?
- If you're growing on a large scale, figure out if you would grow or buy spawn. Both are great options depending upon what your objectives are.

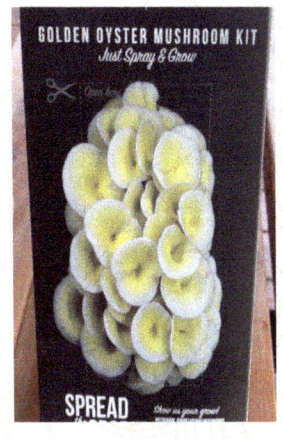

Beginner's Grow Kit   Grow Bag

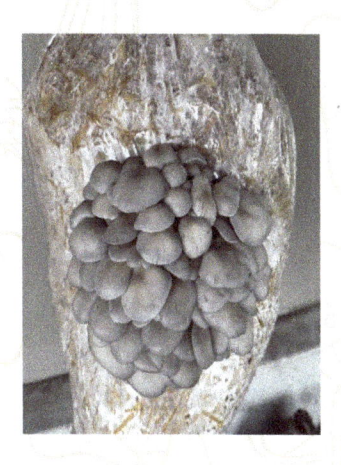

2. I am a newbie lost in a multitude of information online. Just tell me where to begin with minimum requirements? Few tips also would be appreciated, like which processes (minimal) I should focus on? Keep reply as short as possible!

- Minimal things do you need to grow mushrooms - Spores, substrate, a kitchen to sterilize everything, and a temp/humidity controlled area to grow.
- You would need patience, cleanliness, and a little bit of substrate to start.
- Check out Fungi Perfecti from Paul Stamets.
- The easiest way to start is by using Grow Kits or Inoculation Grow Bags.
- Always start with Oyster Mushrooms as they have plenty of information present online.

3. What is the best-supplemented substrate for Turkey Tail and Reishi?

- Hardwood. I supplement reishi with Timothy hay or beet pulp about 10%. Turkey's tails seem to prefer growing everywhere.
- Hardwood sawdust pellets. Add water.

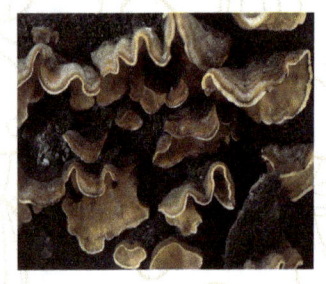

Turkey Tail

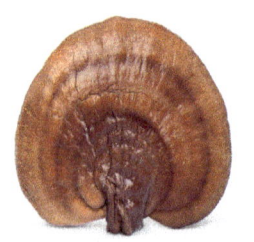

Reishi

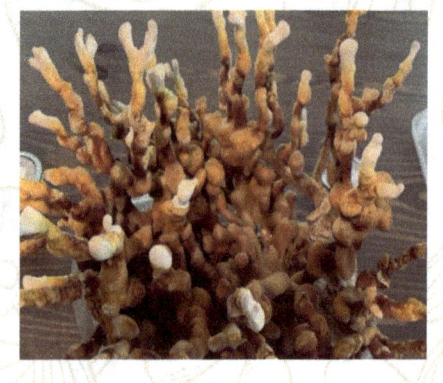

Reishi with Timothy hay or beet pulp

4. I was wondering what happens if we maintain high humidity like in the upper 90's. What impact do it have on mushroom growth and fruiting?

- Though it depends on the mushroom type, you will get bacterial blotch, mutations, and pinning on the caps.
- I swing from 92 down to 80; there is a setting on inkbird (Temperature & Humidity Controller brand), but usually, the temps are low 60s

5. Lots of growers talk about using pasteurized straw in 5-gallon buckets to grow oysters. Is there a reason not to sterilize the straw in a pressure canner? So, for a home grower like me, going for maximum success rate would it help?

- That talk about "full sterilization isn't good for open-air grows" is not correct as I have experienced. What they mean is high nutrient substrates that require full sterilization won't work well in open-air grows. Straw in your pressure cooker is totally fine.

- There is no reason you can't run straight thru the sterilizer. Once I took mushroom cultivation class, they told us they had recently started sterilizing all straw kits they sold to reduce contamination rates. Not sure if they still do, but the few times I did it, it worked just fine.

- Oysters are very aggressive colonizers, and cold water pasteurized straw works very well. Sterilizing is a waste of time.

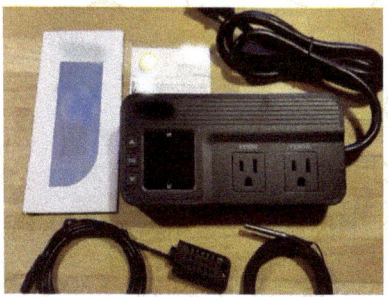

Temperature & Humidity Controller

Substrate used :
- lime pasteurized straw
- lime pasteurized chopped bramble branches
- hot water pasteurized straw pellet

6. After making the batch of agar mix, and once it cools off, we are ready to transfer to the dishes. Below are the queries:

In case we don't have enough dishes for creation, where do we keep the rest? In the refrigerator?

Once we transfer what needs to be inoculated (tissues, spores, LC), where and how to keep them?

You can save your unused agar in the jar. It needs to be sterilized again since it's been opened now—the sterilized agar can be stored either at room temperature or in a refrigerator. You can store liquid culture and swabs at room temp and syringes in the refrigerator.

Agar plates will continue to feed the mycelium until the agar loses pigmentation. That's the clue to know that nutrition has run out. If you're going to keep an agar plate with mycelium on it for a long time, store it in the fridge, that'll slow the growth, and the nutrition will take longer to run out.

If you plan to work with your colonized agar (make transfers) frequently, then you can store it at room temp. Store upside down so condensation doesn't drip on your agar or mycelium.

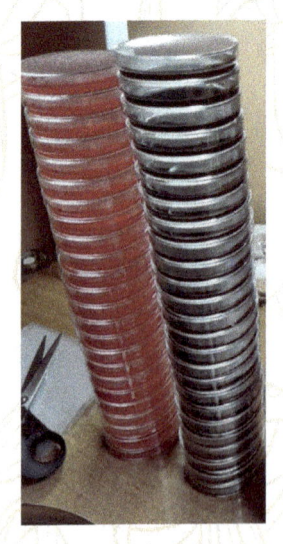

Agar Plates

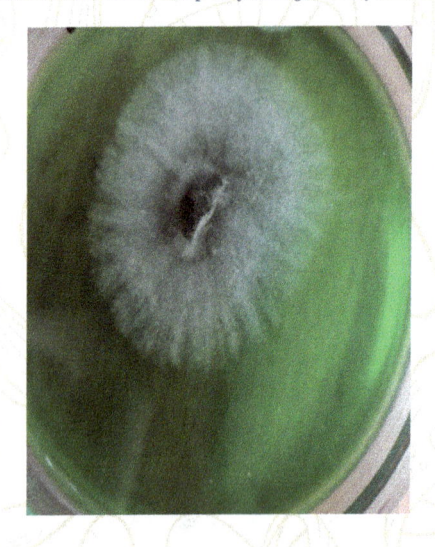

Mycelium from inoculated dowels on T-Gel agar

7. I am a beginner and have raised Blue Oyster mushrooms on a straw grow bag, as shown below. One flush has been harvested. Should I wait for more, or soak in water and try again.

Normally the second flush should start showing in about 3-6 days, should be ready to harvest in 7-12 days, depending on conditions.

You just need to just high humid environment—no need to soak it at this stage.

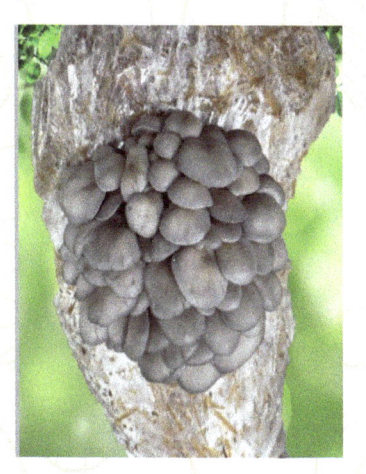

Blue Oyster in Grow Bag

8. I am a beginner and plans to set up a small grow tent. What type of mushrooms is suggest for a beginner.

Any oyster mushrooms. It is colonized in 10-14 days and fruit within a week. The exception being king oysters. It takes four weeks to colonize and two weeks to fruit, plus you'd need an air-conditioned room below 65f.

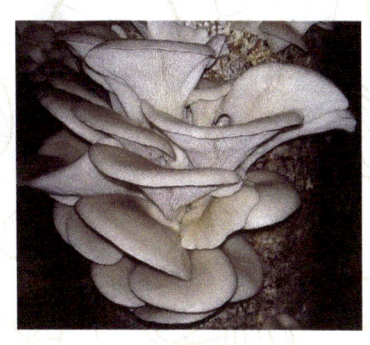

Oyster Mushrooms in Grow Tent White Oyster Harvesting

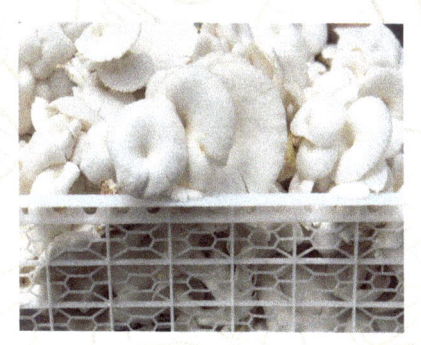

9 . I am a beginner and have some questions regarding inoculating logs. Temperature is moderate in my area (short snow spells).

Can I inoculate trees that are downed for a year or so?

Also, can I inoculate just before fall begins, or is spring the right time?

The appropriate time to cut the trees is late winter. Post that, let them sit for a couple of weeks, then inoculate. It is also important to match the species of mushrooms to the proper species of trees.

In the case of old down logs, they will already have indigenous fungus growing in them, and your inoculation may fail

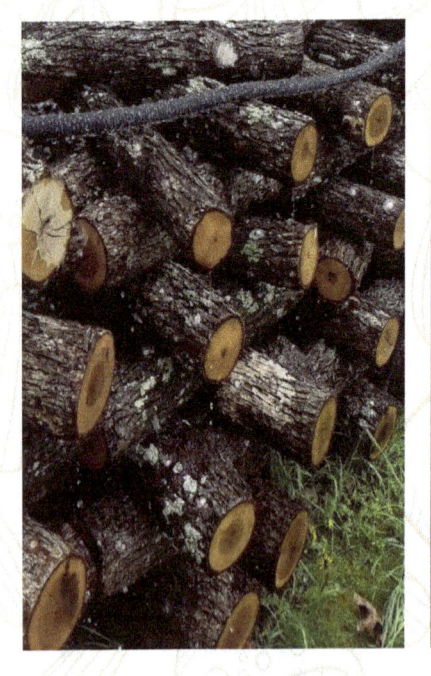

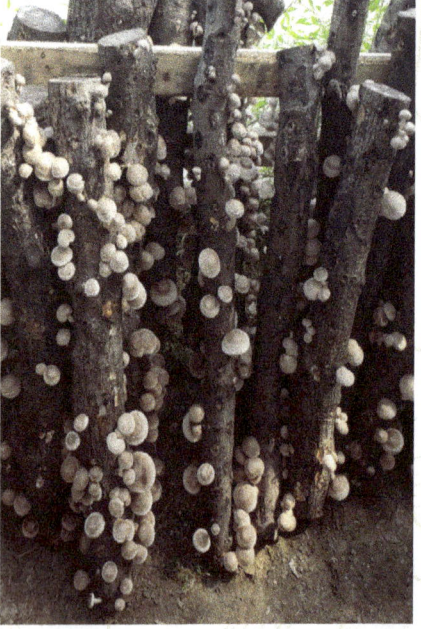

Fresh Logs   Fruiting

10. I am struggling to sell my mushrooms and, as a result, end up with lots of unsold mushrooms. Any tips?

There were multiple solutions suggested for the same. Below is the list of the most relevant ones:

- Try out farmers' markets first; a booth is a great way to meet cooks. Always add a business card with every purchase that links to your social media. As a bonus, you can even give out a recipes booklet with major/long-term sales.
- In case your area is not used to consuming Mushrooms, you can make a pretty basket and provide free samples to restaurants and stores. Follow-up is also important. Visit the same places in some gaps so that they would have feedback.
- Always give a try to high-end restaurants. Make sure to meet the Chef as she/he would be most interested in adding one more specialty dish.
- Make an Instagram and Facebook profile for your Mushroom Store. You can also learn about Facebook ads to target relevant customers in your area. The "Healthy Food " stores, restaurants would be your ideal customer avatar.
- If you have an Asian locality, that would be a certain place where Mushrooms would be consumed. Try selling there.
- An unsold mushroom can be dried out or powdered. Keep stock of your powdered stockpile. You can also make an umami base for stews, stocks, and also vegan sauce. Also, you can make mushroom hamburgers. There are so many means to utilize the leftover mushroom.
- Dehydrate and sell online.

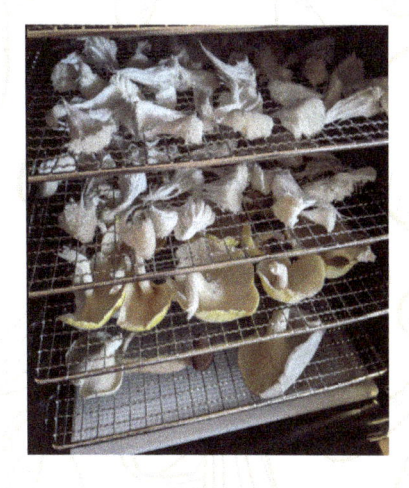

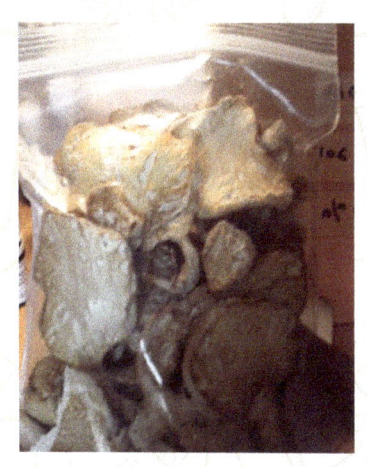

Dehydrator

Dried Mushroom

9. Conclusion

I want to thank you once again for choosing this book. I hope it proved to be an enjoyable and informative read.

In this book, you were introduced to pretty much everything you need to know about cultivating mushrooms at home. Depending on the mushroom species and the growing conditions, they come in a variety of shapes, sizes, and colors. A wonderful thing about growing mushrooms at home is it gives you complete control over not just the types you want to grow but how much to grow and how you grow them.

This flexibility will make it easier to grow different types of mushrooms within no time. All it requires is a little patience, the willingness to go through the learning curve involved in this process, effort, and consistency. Once you are willing to make this commitment, cultivating mushrooms at home will become incredibly simple.

Now that you have gone through all the information in this book, you will have realized that cultivating mushrooms at home is no harder than growing any other common plant. This is not only an enjoyable activity that can be transformed into a hobby but can be used to create an additional source of income. Use the business ideas and advice to set up a side hustle by cultivating mushrooms at home.

So, what are you waiting for?

All the information you need to get started with cultivating mushrooms at home has been given to you. All that's left for you to do now is select a type of mushroom you want to grow, use the growing techniques discussed in this book, and get started. Once you get the hang of it, you can also transform this hobby or interest into a side hustle! So get started immediately to reap all the benefits associated with growing mushrooms at home.

Thank you and all the best!

Stephen Fleming

10. Glossary

Agar in Mushrooming

Agar is utilized in the cultivation of mushrooms in order to save cultures for long-lasting use and save them from being contaminated. Spores are germinated on agar before clean transfer to the new agar plate.

Martha Chamber:

The Martha chamber is named after Martha Stewart, who made a hanging closet. It is referred to as basically any small-sized zip-curtained mushroom fruiting chamber which has shelves, a synthetic, non-porous cover to retain humidity.

HWFP - Hardwood fuel pellets

Available at most hardware or feed stores, it is mostly used in pellet stoves for heating. In mushrooming, it is one of the most convenient and standard fruiting substrates that produce good results.

SBH - Soybean hull (typically pellets)

A Frequently made use of as animals feed. Part of many preferred fruiting substrate formulas in conjunction with hardwood fuel pellets.

Lime

Normally, when people discuss lime, they indicate hydrated lime (calcium hydroxide.) As long as it's calcium hydroxide and has low magnesium, it's okay.

Lipa

Refers to a strategy of pasteurizing fuel pellets with boiling water and keeping them protected, so they preserve their warmth long enough to be pasteurized.

PC - Pressure cooker/ pressure canner.

A pressure vessel, generally utilized on a stovetop, can reach as well as keep 15 PSI.

PDYA/PDA/MEA/ MEYA/etc.

These mostly refer to agar recipes. PDA is potato dextrose agar, PDYA is potato dextrose yeast agar, MEA is malt extract agar, and so forth. Agar recipes generally contain the agar itself, which are added nutrients and various other substances to motivate mycelium growth.

LME

Light malt extract. Utilized for making agar solutions and also frequently likewise utilized for liquid culture broth.

GE

Gas Exchange. Describes the slow diffusion of gases through a filter medium of some kind (filter spot, firmly packed poly loading, and so on) while mycelium is colonizing. Not to be confused with FAE.

FAE

Fresh air exchange. Much more than a gas exchange, this describes the constant fresh air exchanges right into the growing area to maintain CO_2 levels and stop stunted mushroom development.

Grow Bags

Unless speaking about straw, this usually refers to gusseted polypropylene bags with a patch of filter material near the top to offer a gas exchange. The filter is usually either 0.5 or 0.2 microns.

Straw log

A section of plastic tubes, normally from a roll, is packed with straw (blended with spawn) and secured. Frequently holes are poked for airflow.

Bucket fogger

A humidity-generating system that usually includes a huge (5 gallon) bucket, an ultrasonic mist manufacturer, a fan, and also some plumbing to relocate the haze to where it's required.

Plugs/plug spawn/dowel spawn

5/16" x 1" dowel pins inoculated with mushroom mycelium. They are generally pounded into holes drilled in appropriate logs as well as sealed over with wax for log-style growing.

Grain spawn

Hydrated, sterilized grains (often rye, yet others are utilized), totally colonized with mycelium. Useful to inoculate fruiting substrates such as sawdust or straw. Not suitable to inoculate logs.

WBS

Wild birdseed. A mixture of millet, wheat, sunflower seeds, as well as others depending on the solution. Corn is normally prevented as a result of ending up being sticky after hydration, in some cases utilized for grain spawn.

Sawdust spawn

Usually a grow bag (see over) full of colonized sawdust. It can be made use of to inoculate outdoor beds, plug logs (a special tool is required), or several types can be fruited straight from sawdust.

SAB

Still-air box. A clear plastic tote (or various other constructed rooms) with two holes for arms yet otherwise confined to reduce air movement and reduce contamination. Not to be confused with a glove box, which has permanently affixed gloves at the arm openings, which can worsen air currents inside the box.

APPENDIX 1 : Process Flow

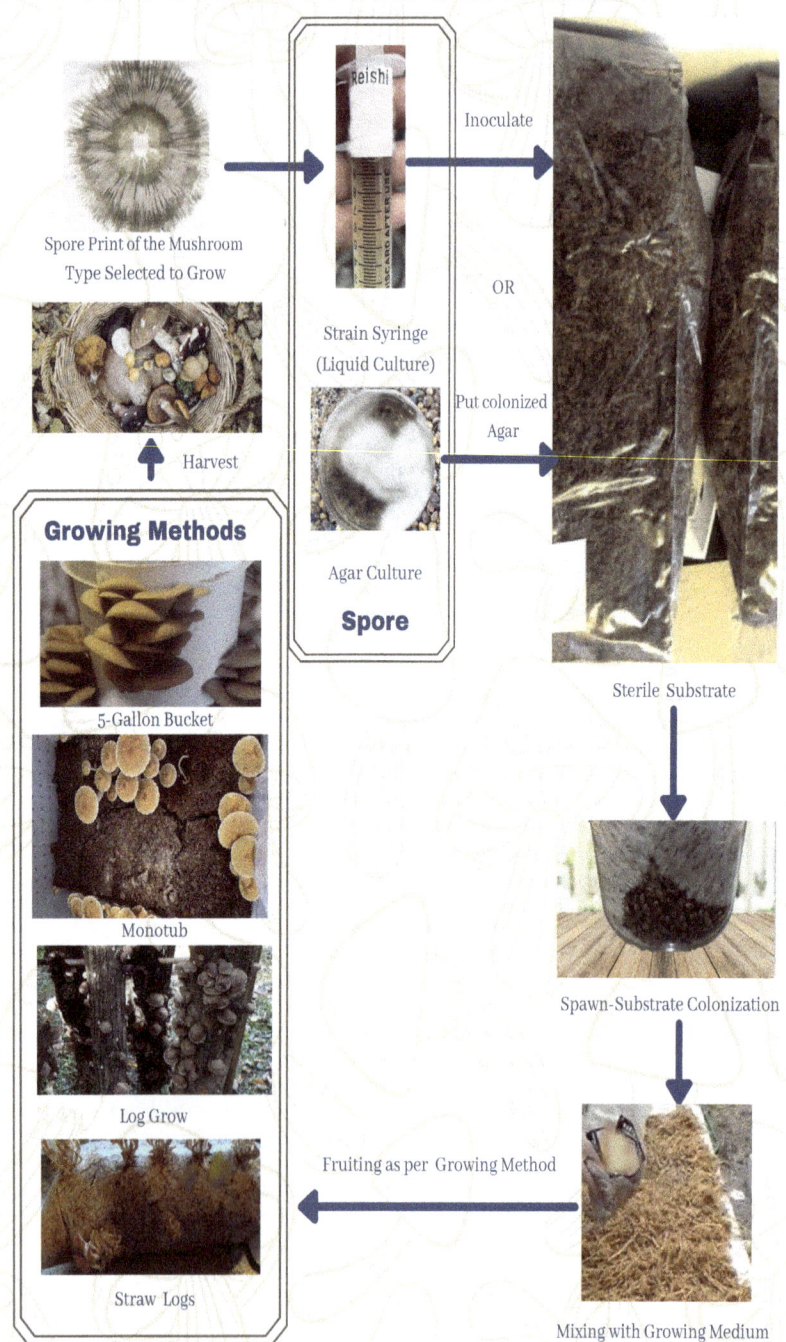

Spore Print of the Mushroom Type Selected to Grow

Harvest

Inoculate

Strain Syringe (Liquid Culture)

OR

Put colonized Agar

Agar Culture

Spore

Sterile Substrate

Spawn-Substrate Colonization

Mixing with Growing Medium

Fruiting as per Growing Method

Growing Methods

5-Gallon Bucket

Monotub

Log Grow

Straw Logs

127

APPENDIX 2 : Precautions

- Fumigate the rooms before making the raising beds. Fumigation includes blending formalin with potassium permanganate and letting the fumes inhabit the whole room.

- Before entering either growing area, we need to clean the hands and legs with soap. Stringent hygienic conditions must be preserved inside as well as properties of the homestead. Do not use a broomstick.

- Constantly keep an eye on the temperature as well as humidity percentages inside the space. Check the contaminants regularly.

-
- Do not permit any outsider in your growing area as humans carry many contaminants detrimental to mushroom growth.

- And finally, have patience and wait for growth.

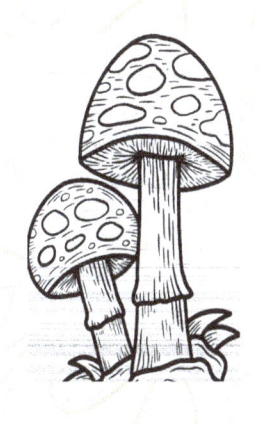

APPENDIX 3 : Mushroom Tree Compatibility

Mushroom Type	Tree Species
Shiitake	Alder,Ash,Beech,Chestnut,Cottonwood,Elm,Eucalyptus,Hickory,Maple,Oaks,Sweetgum
Oyster	Alder,Beech,Birch,Poplar,Elm,Maple,Oaks
Nameko	Alder,Maple,Oaks
Lion's Mane	Chestnut,Poplar/Cottonwood,Elm,Maple,Oaks
Reishi	Poplar/Cottonwood,Elm,Maple,Oaks
Chicken of Woods	Fir,Hemlock,Spruce
Turkey Tail	Alder,Ash,Beech,Chestnut,Cottonwood,Elm,Eucalyptus,Hickory,Maple,Oaks,Sweetgum,Birch,Elm,Fir,Hemlocks,Spruce,Plum,Magnolia,Honey Locust,Willow,Tupelo,Ironwood
Maitake	Poplar,Elm,Honey Locust,Maple,Oaks
King Oyester	Oaks

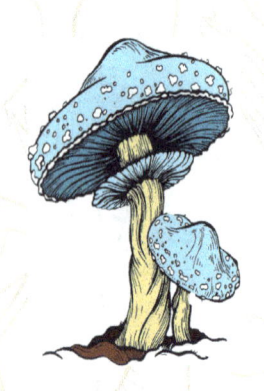

We'd Love Your Feedback!

★ ★ ★ ★ ★

Please let us know how we're doing by leaving us a review.

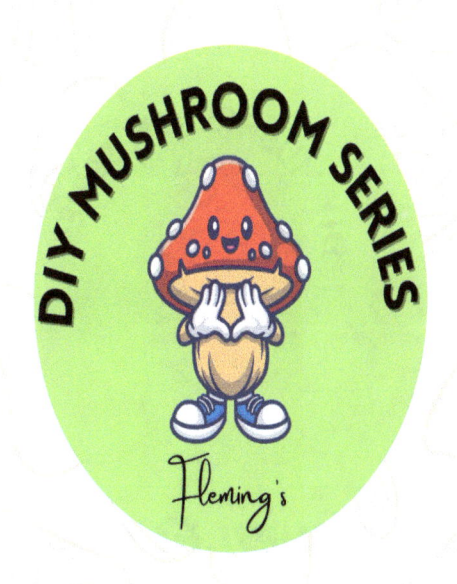

DIY MUSHROOM SERIES
Fleming's

MR. FLEMING'S

THE MEDICINAL MUSHROOM STARTER HANDBOOK

18 Healing Mushrooms, Foraging & Usage Tips. Recipes & FAQ's

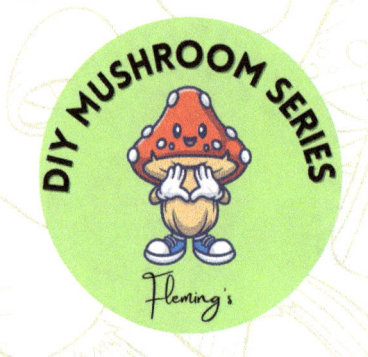

Stephen Fleming

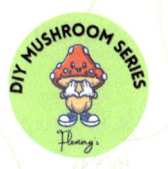

© Copyright 2021 - All rights reserved.

The content contained within this book may not be reproduced, duplicated or transmitted without direct written permission from the author or the publisher.

Under no circumstances will any blame or legal responsibility be held against the publisher, or author, for any damages, reparation, or monetary loss due to the information contained within this book, either directly or indirectly.

Legal Notice:
This book is copyright protected. It is only for personal use. You cannot amend, distribute, sell, use, quote, or paraphrase any part, or the content within this book, without the author or publisher's consent.

Disclaimer Notice:
Please note the information contained within this document is for educational and entertainment purposes only. All effort has been executed to present accurate, up-to-date, reliable, complete information. No warranties of any kind are declared or implied. Readers acknowledge that the author is not engaged in the rendering of legal, financial, medical or professional advice. The content within this book has been derived from various sources. Please consult a licensed professional before attempting any techniques outlined in this book.

By reading this document, the reader agrees that under no circumstances is the author responsible for any losses, direct or indirect, that are incurred as a result of the use of the information contained within this document, including, but not limited to, errors, omissions, or inaccuracies.

Disclaimer

- The objective of the book is simply to provide information; it is not intended to replace diagnosis and treatment, tasks which pertain to a doctor.

- The contents of this book are for informational & educational purposes and are not intended to offer personal medical advice.

- You should seek the advice of your physician or another qualified health provider regarding a medical condition. Never disregard professional medical advice or delay seeking it because of something you have read in this book. The book does not recommend or endorse any products.

- Any book, video, or other means of learning can't replace learning physically from an expert. These forms of information are only additional guidance to be used along with a practical demonstration and training.

- Always check the legal status of the mushroom you intend to grow and use.

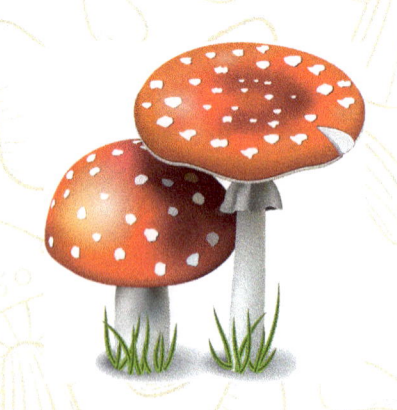

Chapters

1. Story of Healing Mushrooms- Otzi the Iceman to Alexander Fleming
2. Let's Meet 18 Medicinal Mushrooms
3. How Mushrooms Heal
4. Identifying/Foraging Top 7 Medicinal Mushrooms
5. How to Take Medicinal Mushrooms
6. How to cook Medicinal Mushrooms: 7 Recipes
7. Frequently Asked Questions (FAQ) & Glossary
8. Conclusion
9. Reference

1. Story of Healing Mushrooms- Otzi the Iceman to Alexander Fleming

Nature alone is antique, and the oldest art a Mushroom
- Thomas Carlyle

Introduction

Mushrooms are incredibly nutritious and have a variety of minerals, vitamins, and beneficial compounds that improve your overall health and wellbeing. From mental to physical health, the benefits offered by mushrooms cannot be overlooked. As a result, medicinal mushrooms have slowly started gaining popularity in recent times.

That said, the medicinal use of mushrooms has been around for a long time and is a long-prevailing tradition across different cultures worldwide. Mushrooms have helped protect humanity's health for hundreds of years. These days, there is a steadily increasing body of scientific evidence that shows the biologically active compounds present in mushrooms offer significant health benefits.

Mushrooms contain some of the most potent and helpful natural medicines known to humans. There are tens of thousands of species of mushrooms, and we are only familiar with about 10% of them.

There are around 270 species of mushrooms believed to have therapeutic properties, and about 100 species are being studied for their health-promoting benefits.

Medicinal mushrooms are among the most priced natural possessions, and they can build and strengthen human health and functioning.

There's a similarity between humans and mushrooms in terms of the pathogens they are exposed to. Fungi have potent antimicrobial defense mechanisms in place to protect themselves from harmful pathogens. Upon consumption of these mushrooms, the highly absorbable medical constituents in them are recognized by the human body and used to strengthen itself from the inside. Did you know that tetracycline, penicillin, and streptomycin are all fungal extracts?

History of Medicinal Mushrooms

The idea of using medicinal mushrooms is not anything new. Humans have been using medicinal mushrooms as part of traditional or folk medicine even before recorded history.

Otzi the Iceman: For instance, mummified remains of a man who is believed to be frozen in ice around 3300 BCE were discovered around the Alps in 1991. This fully preserved specimen had two different species of mushrooms with him!

One fungus was a medicinal polypore mushroom that is commonly used for fighting infections and other pathogens. The other mushroom he was holding was a Tinder fungus used to fire in ancient times.

Archaeologists also discovered ancient Egyptian hieroglyphics that showcase the critical role played by mushrooms.

In ancient Egypt, only Pharaohs and other nobles were allowed to eat mushrooms, and they were believed to be the sons of the gods.

Some artwork discovered by archaeologists shows mushrooms were considered as gifts given by the almighty sent to earth in the form of lightning worlds.

Famous Greek and Roman thinkers and authors from ancient Egypt unknown to have argued for and against the medicinal properties and benefits offered by mushrooms.

The list includes some famous names such as Pliny, Dioscorides, and Seneca. There's also Chinese text dating back to 100 BCE showing how mushrooms were used for treating a variety of problems including respiratory ailments.

For instance, Reishi mushrooms have the longest known history when it comes to their medicinal usage. However, science is only now beginning to understand how wonderful medicinal mushrooms genuinely are and their potential.

So here is a fun fact about mushroom history- Maitake mushrooms were used as currency that too equivalent to the silver weight in ancient Japan!

In addition, mushrooms were also an essential part of indigenous Mesoamerican cultures such as the Aztecs, Mayans, Incas, and Olmecs.

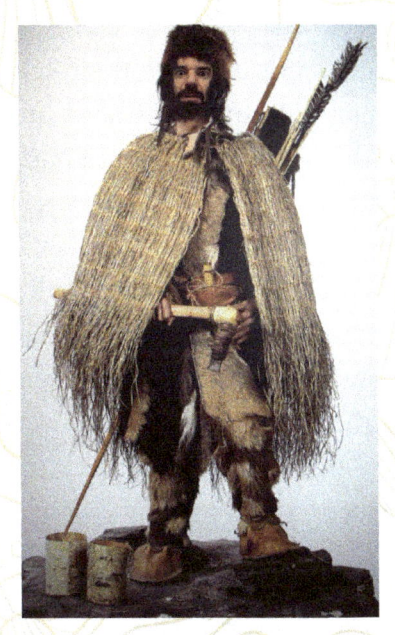

Otzi the Iceman - Reconstruction
Attribution: By Melotzi - Own work, CC BY-SA 4.0,
https://commons.wikimedia.org/w/index.php?curid=64153648

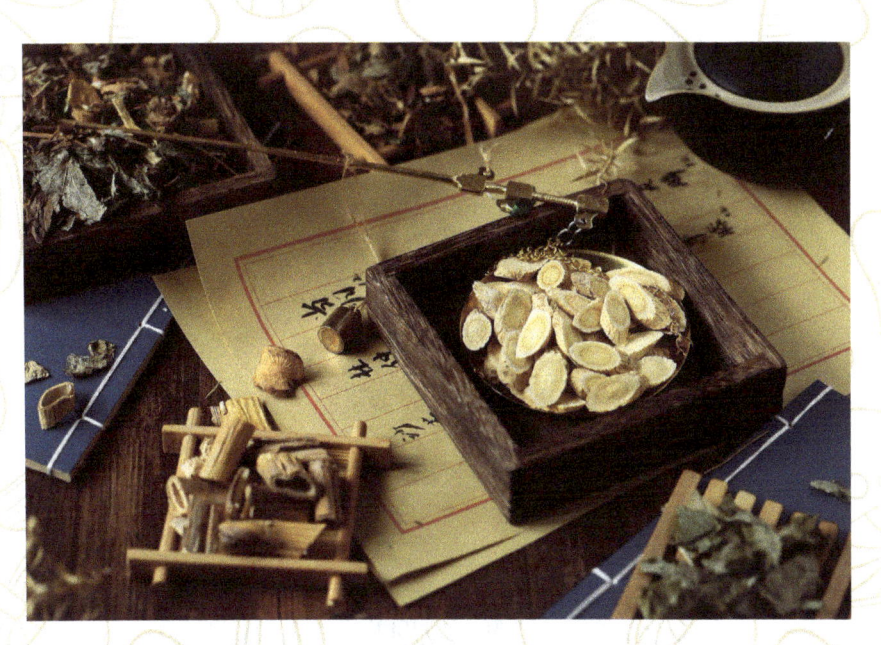

Traditional Chinese Herbal Medicine

These beautiful fungi were used for their spiritual and healing properties by shamans. Records of Chaga and other medicinal mushrooms being used across Siberia and northern America date back to the 16th century.

The history of medicinal mushrooms and their usage isn't restricted to ancient times. You might have heard that Alexander Fleming was responsible for discovering penicillin, a common antibacterial drug that revolutionized the world of science and medicine!

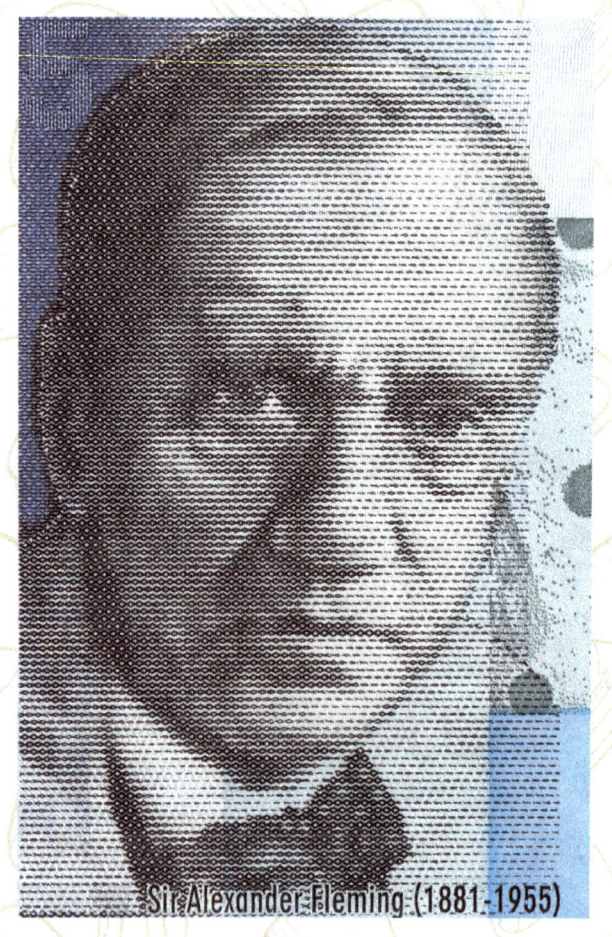

Sir Alexander Fleming (1881-1955)

Alexander Fleming

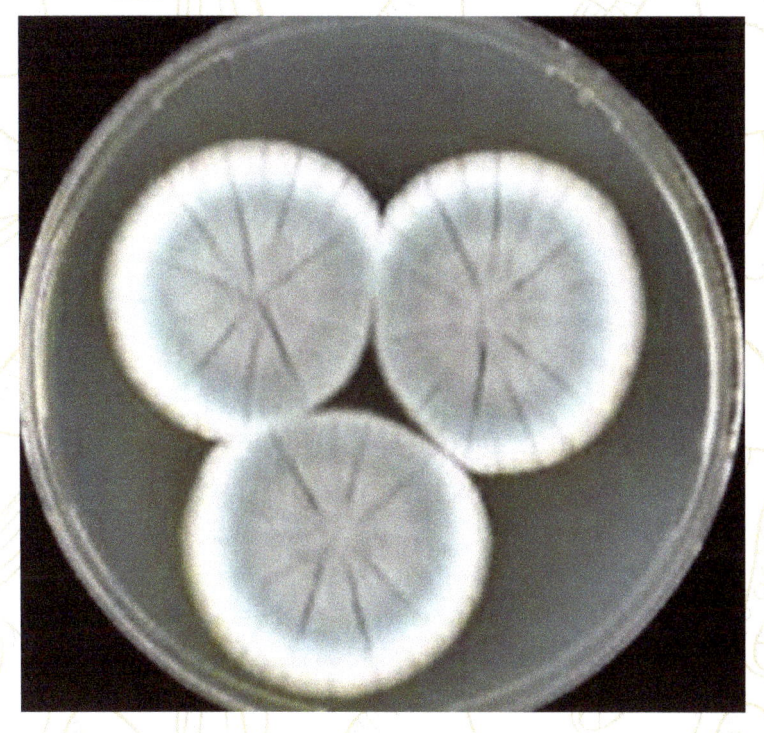

Penicillin Specimen

Attribution: Houbraken, J., Frisvad, J.C. & Samson, R.A, CC BY-SA 4.0 <https://creativecommons.org/licenses/by-sa/4.0>, via Wikimedia Commons

Fleming created this drug from a type of fungus known as penicillin. Modern scientists are still trying to isolate the healing, anti-microbial, and immune-boosting properties of different fungi.

Likewise, scientists, including mycologists, are only now exploring mushrooms' immense healing and medicinal potential that traditional medicine has been using for thousands of years now.

2. Let's Meet 18 Medicinal Mushrooms

The sudden appearance of mushrooms after a summer rain is one of the more impressive spectacles of the plant world.
- John Tyler Bonner

Learning about different types of medicinal mushrooms and their medicinal properties will increase your appreciation for these humble fungi.

1. Agaricus Bisporus (Cremini mushrooms, Button mushrooms, & Portobello)

The Agaricus bisporus species of mushrooms include a variety of common mushrooms such as Cremini mushrooms, Button mushrooms, and Portobello. These mushrooms are quite popular and consumed globally. All the varieties included in this species are perfectly edible and also have medicinal properties.

The freshest and the youngest of the species are known as white button mushrooms. Once they mature for a while, they turn into cremini mushrooms. When they are left for the longest period and fully mature, they turn into Portobello mushrooms.

Button mushrooms are usually bright white-colored while cremini has a brownish color and Portobello mushrooms are dark brown colored. All these mushrooms are low in calories, contain helpful fiber, are a rich source of protein, and don't have any harmful fats in them.

These mushrooms are also rich in a variety of antioxidants and have immune-boosting properties too. Apart from this, these mushrooms are believed to prevent the hardening of arteries, fight type-2 diabetes, improve liver health and reduce cholesterol levels. They are also associated with better cardiovascular health, reduction of stomach ulcers, and healthier bones.

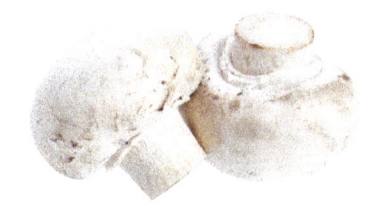

Button Mushroom

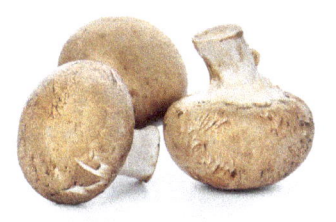

Cremini Mushroom

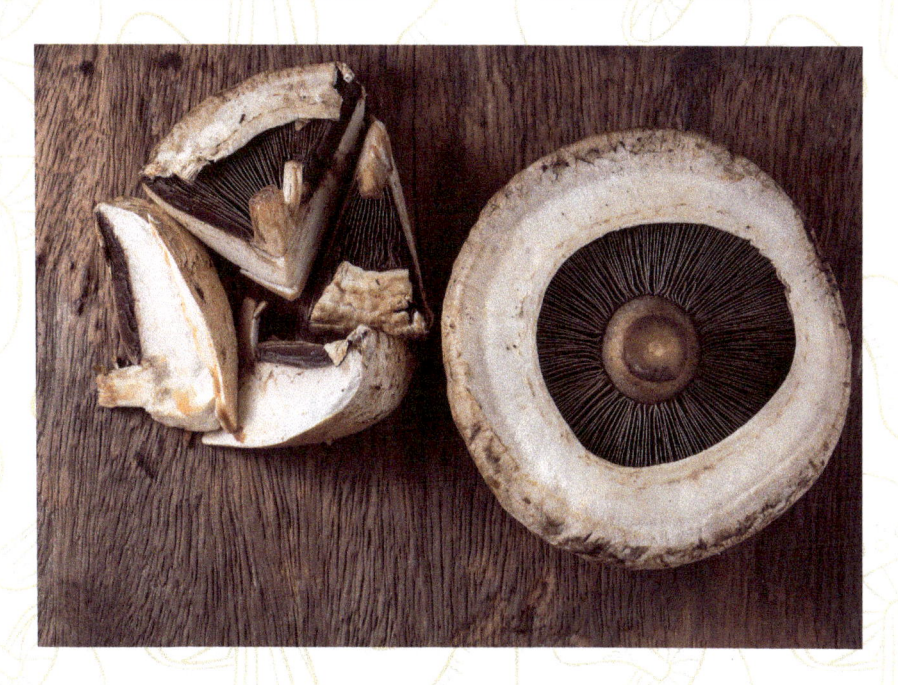

Portobello Mushroom

2. Boletus Edulis (Porcini)

You must be aware of this mushroom if you are interested in Italian and French recipes.

Still, wondering what this mushroom is?

Well, it's nothing but porcini!

These earthy and wonderful mushrooms can instantly elevate the flavor profile of any pasta or risotto you want to cook. It has an early taste with a reddish cap. They are rich in a compound known as Ergosterol, responsible for enhancing your body's ability to fight cellular infections.

The antioxidants present in it also regulate your body's inflammatory response.

All in all, these mushrooms are good for improving the functioning of the immune system. A more robust immune system automatically reduces your susceptibility to infections.

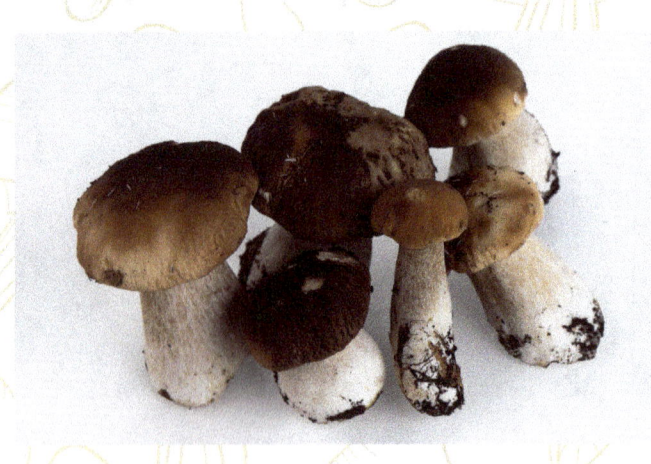

Boletus Edulis or Porcini Mushroom

3. Cordyceps Militaris

These mushrooms are commonly known as Cordyceps and are quite popular in traditional Chinese medicine.

It has several antioxidants, and its antiviral and antibacterial properties make it a truly remarkable mushroom.

The tincture is made with Cordyceps and can improve liver and kidney health, promote better blood circulation, treat asthma, and reduce blood pressure levels.

It is believed to improve athletic performance, tackle diabetes, fight certain types of cancer, and even treat sexual dysfunction in men.

They are also used to improve cognitive functioning and brain health. As long as you don't have any bleeding disorders such as sickle cell disease or hemophilia and are not scheduled for surgery soon, these mushrooms are safe.

It is a successful commercially cultivated species in an artificial environment.

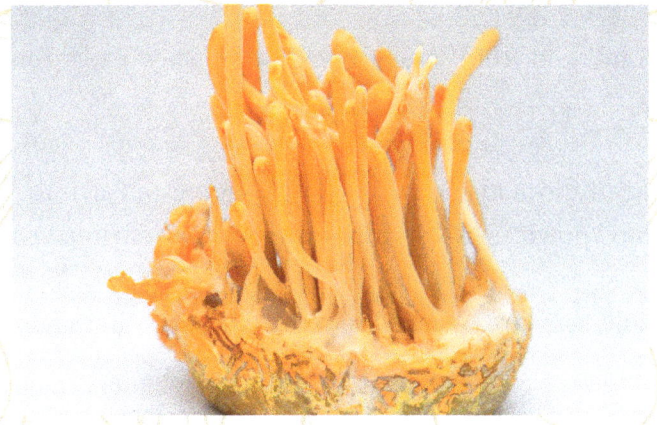

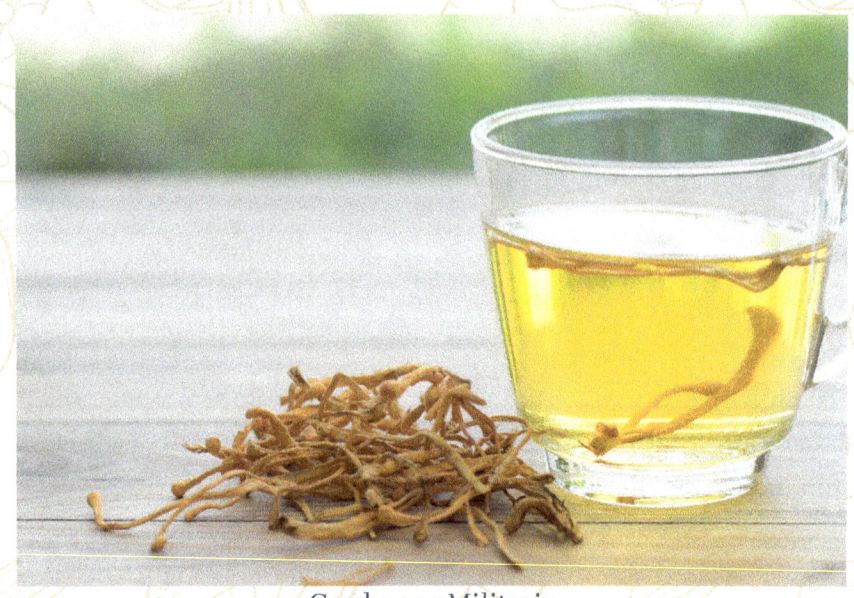

Cordyceps Militaris

4. Flammulina Velutipes(Enoki)

The common name of these mushrooms is Enokitake mushrooms, also known as enoki.

These mushrooms are incredibly popular in East Asian countries like China, Japan, Vietnam, and Korea. They are also commonly used in Asian cooking.

These long and thin mushrooms with tiny caps resemble noodles!

A helpful amino acid known as Ergothioneine and an anti-tumor compound known as prolamin are present in these mushrooms.

As a result, they are believed to reduce the risk of certain types of cancer.

Enoki mushrooms also support and strengthen the functioning of the immune system and improve your body's ability to fight off infections and disease-causing pathogens.

They also help regulate the levels of LDL, which reduces the risk of atherosclerosis. This, in turn, can improve your cardiovascular health. Regular consumption of enoki can improve your digestive health and metabolism too.

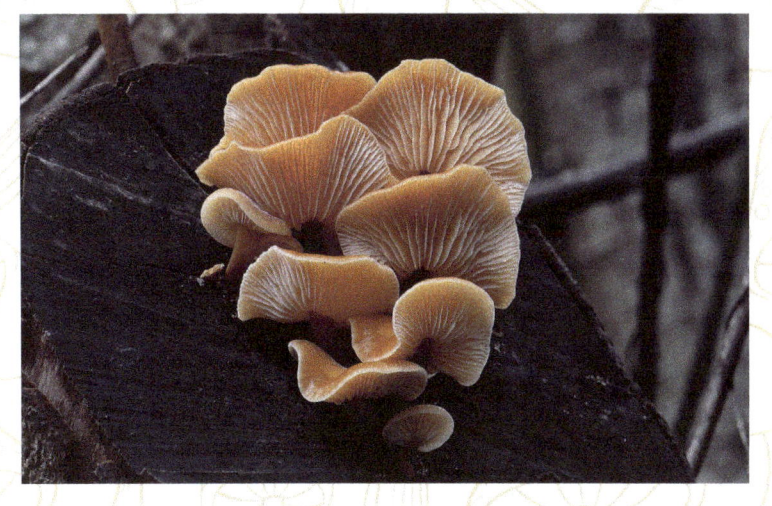

Wild enokitake

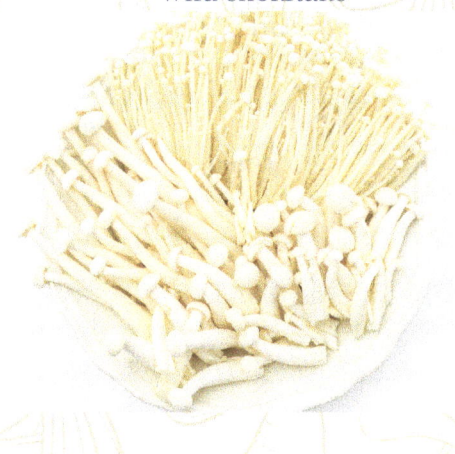

Cultivated enokitake or Golden Needle

5. Fomitopsis Betulina (Birch Polypore)

The common name of this mushroom is birch polypore. These mushrooms are named so because they are commonly found on Birch trees.

They're known as razor strop fungus too. They are native to the northern hemisphere and are commonly found in Asia, Northern America, and Europe.

It has a long and exciting history of medicinal uses. Initially, a tincture made with these mushrooms was used by barbers to wipe their razors. They were also used as an emery board for polishing metals. Apart from these interesting uses, polypore also has several medical applications. Some helpful compounds present in them include piptamine, betulinic acid, and triterpene acid.

These mushrooms can help strengthen your immune function and have several anti-fungal, anti-viral, and antibacterial properties. They are also believed to reduce inflammation.

They also have antiseptic properties; apart from this, the beneficial compounds mentioned above destroy tumor cells without harming the healthy ones.

Therefore, they are believed to fight certain types of cancers and tumors.

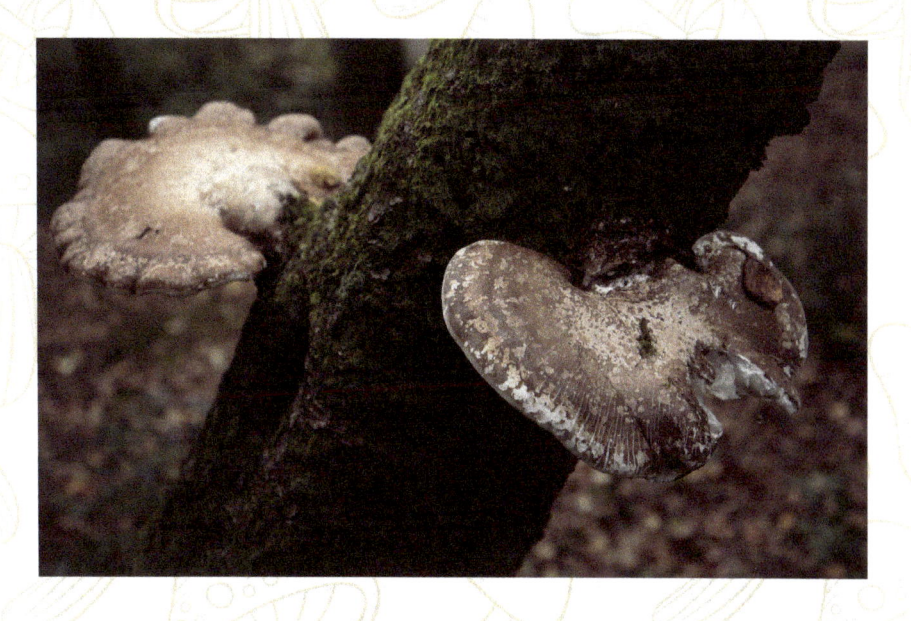

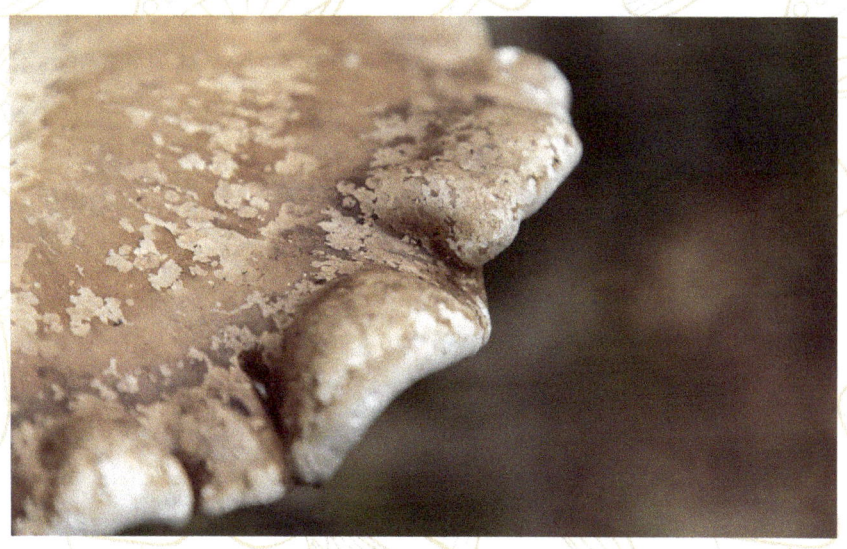

Birch Polypore

6. Ganoderma Lucidum (Reishi)

The reishi mushroom or Ganoderma lucidum is one of the most popular mushrooms, and it is commonly used as an herbal remedy by different cultures across the world.

It is an apoptogenic fungus and is dubbed as the mushroom of immortality because it helps various health problems. This mushroom has a lot to offer, from tackling inflammation to repairing damaged vessels, reducing allergy symptoms, treating hormonal imbalances, elevating energy levels, and even fighting cancer and infections.

A tincture made with these mushrooms will help regulate and strengthen immune functioning while reducing the presence of free radicals responsible for inflammation and oxidative stress.

Some health problems such as rheumatoid arthritis, inflammatory disorders, multiple sclerosis, lupus, and other conditions triggered by stress can be kept at bay by using reishi tinctures.

These mushrooms are also believed to help regulate blood sugar and cholesterol levels while improving cardiovascular health. Heart functioning and blood pressure can also be stabilized by using these mushrooms regularly.

These beautiful mushrooms also have certain neuroprotective effects. Since they help tackle inflammation and improve immune response, they can also help treat leaky gut or irritable bowel syndrome.

Never consume these mushrooms if you have any bleeding disorders such as sickle cell disease or hemophilia. Apart from this, don't use them if you are scheduled to undergo surgery soon.

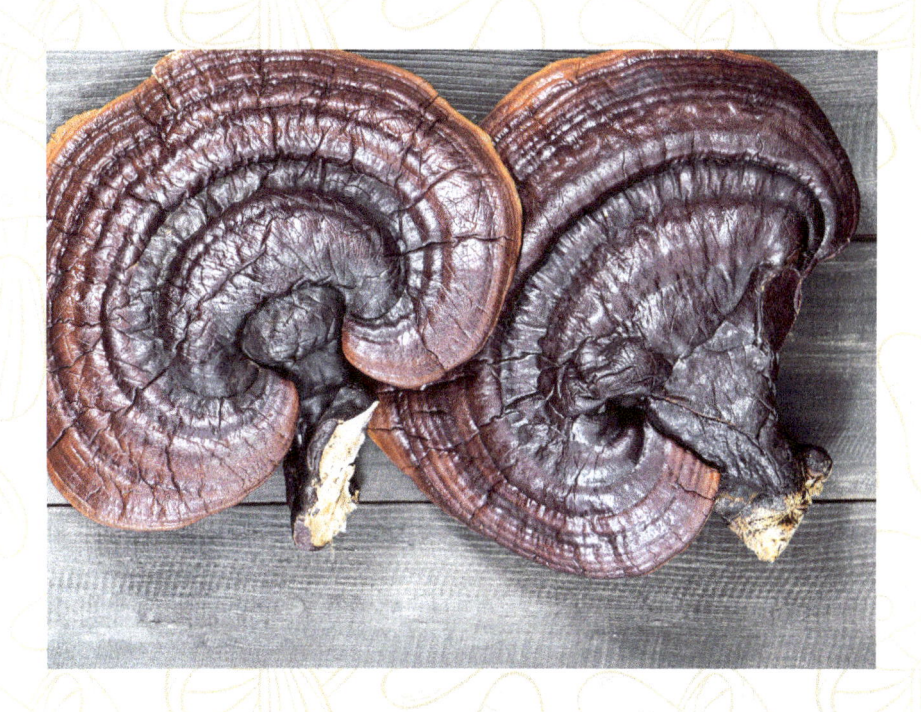

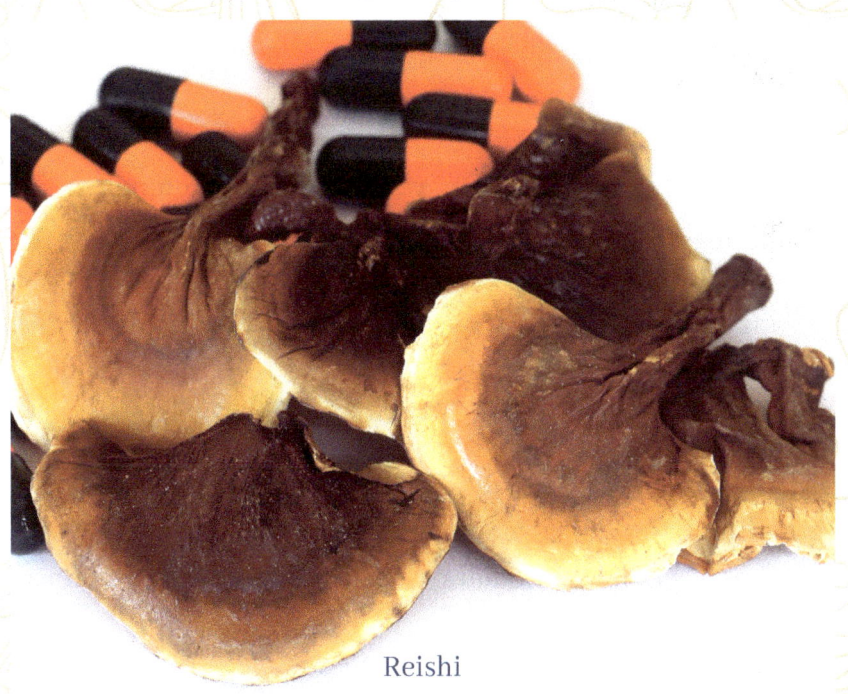

Reishi

7. Hericium Erinaceus (Lion's Mane)

These mushrooms are popularly known as the lion's mane. They are not only medicinal mushrooms but are one of the most sought-after edible ones as well.

These unique mushrooms offer a variety of health benefits. They are usually sought after for their ability to deal with neurodegenerative conditions such as multiple sclerosis, Alzheimer's, and Parkinson's. The proteins responsible for nerve regeneration become more active upon consumption of the specific mushroom tincture.

Other psychological issues such as stress-related disorders, mood disorders, including depression and anxiety, can also be treated with it.

Hericenones and erinacines are the dominant components of this mushroom and are responsible for improving nerve repair. A combination of all these factors strengthens the health of the nervous system and prevents or reduces the risk of neurodegeneration.

Apart from this, the antioxidant and anti-inflammatory properties of the lion's mane mushroom are shown to have a positive effect on gut inflammation. This, in turn, strengthens gut health.

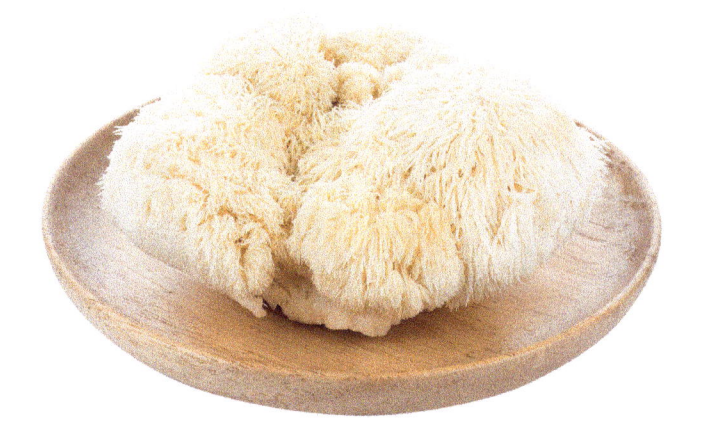

Lion's Mane

8. Inonotus Obliquus (Chaga Mushroom)

One of the most famous & helpful medicinal mushrooms known is the Chaga mushroom. These mushrooms are beneficial, from reducing the accumulation of free radicals responsible for oxidative damage to improving your overall health.

It's commonly consumed in the form of tea. The high levels of polyphenols present in them strengthen immune functioning while tackling inflammation.

Apart from this, if you are dealing with high blood pressure, high cholesterol, and diabetes, these mushrooms will come in handy.

Furthermore, since these mushrooms help rectify the health markers associated with cardiovascular diseases, your heart's health will also improve.

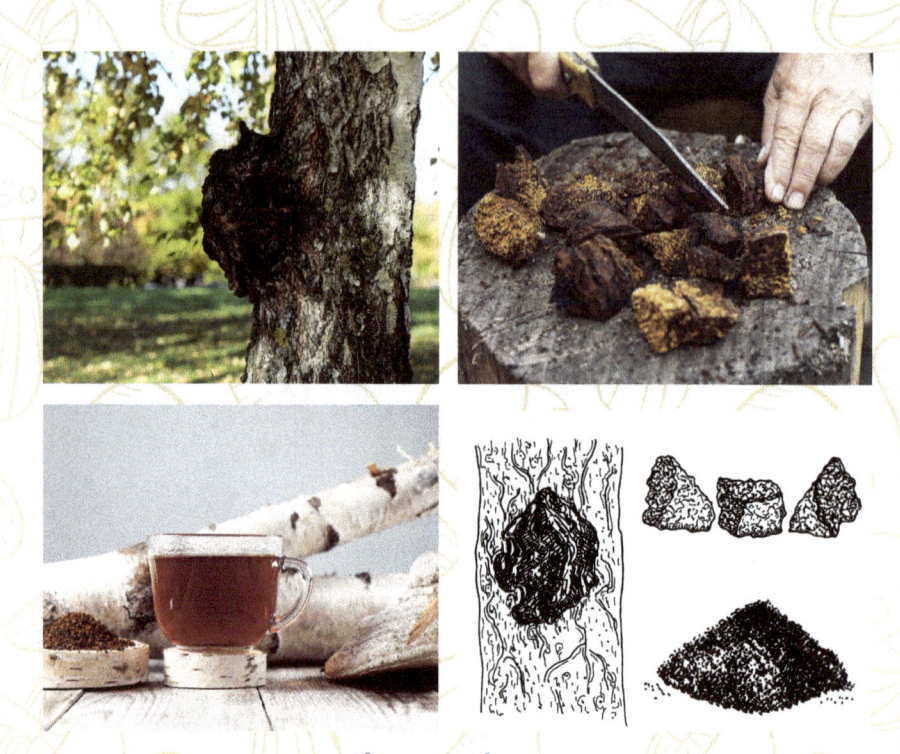

Chaga Mushroom

9. Grifola Frondosa (Maitake Mushroom)

The scientific name of maitake mushrooms is Grifola Frondosa. These mushrooms are rich in dietary fibers and are believed to help regulate blood sugar levels. They are also an adaptogen that comes in handy, especially in patients with diabetes, because of their insulin resistance-enhancing properties.

Apart from this, these incredible mushrooms enhance your immune system's ability to tackle various disease-causing microbes and pathogens.

If you are looking for a better ability to manage the stress you experience and regain balance between your mental and physical wellbeing, then using these mushrooms will come in handy.

Vitamin C, beta-glucans, niacin, and a variety of other essential nutrients are found in these mushrooms. The occurrence of malignancy can be reduced by regularly using maitake extracts.

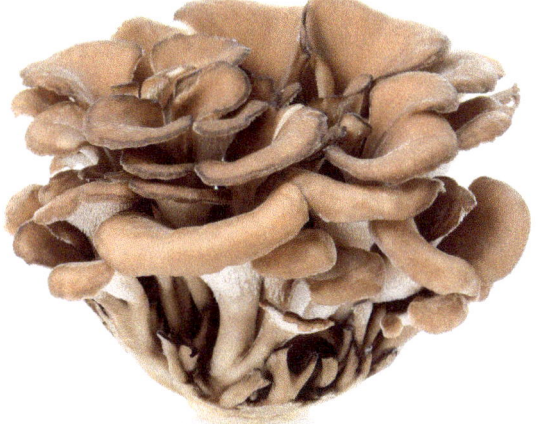

Maitake Mushroom

10. Trametes Versicolor (Turkey Tail)

The scientific name of the Turkey Tail mushroom is Trametes Versicolor. As with most of the other mushrooms common, even this specific variety is rich in essential vitamins, polysaccharides, and beta-glucans.

These are responsible for regulating immune functioning as well as improving digestive health. The prebiotic fibers present in the turkey tail mushroom will help restore and improve digestive processes.

These mushrooms can be used for improving gastric motility, preventing bacterial overgrowth and small understanding, and reducing the risk of a leaky gut. This mushroom is also believed to have certain cancer-fighting properties and is commonly used in conjunction with pharmaceutical treatments for cancer.

It's also known for its immune modulation properties. Tinctures made with the turkey tail mushroom are used for treating ailments such as inflammation, herpes, influenza, and even human papillomavirus (HPV).

You can use the tea extracts made with it, but this only gives you water-soluble compounds, while you can obtain the full spectrum of all the medicinal benefits it offers by using a dual extracted tincture from these mushrooms.

You can use the tea extracts made with it, but this only gives you water-soluble compounds, while you can obtain the full spectrum of all the medicinal benefits it offers by using a dual extracted tincture from these mushrooms.

Lowering bad cholesterol, Slowing Aging, Anti-Inflammation

Turkey Tail

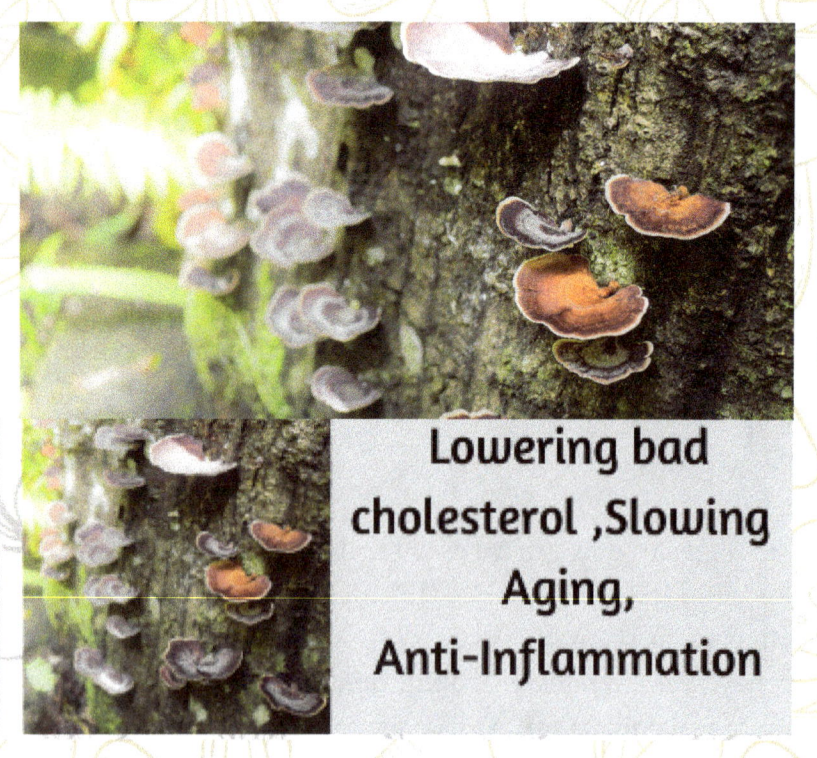

11. Lentinula Edodes (Shiitake Mushroom)

Don't get scared looking at the scientific name because they are commonly known as shiitake mushrooms. These edible mushrooms have a rich flavor making them quite sought after, especially in Asian cooking.

They are believed to have immunity-boosting functions and anti-microbial properties.

The high levels of vitamin D present in them promote bone and tooth health while improving your body's ability to absorb calcium.

They also have an anti-tumor compound known as Lentinan that prevents the growth of benign tumors.

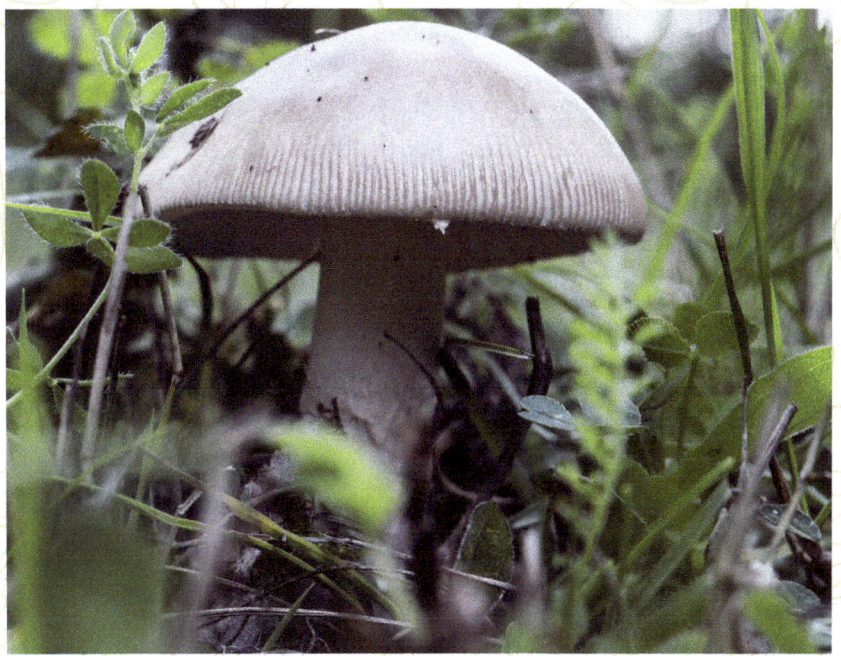

Shiitake in nature

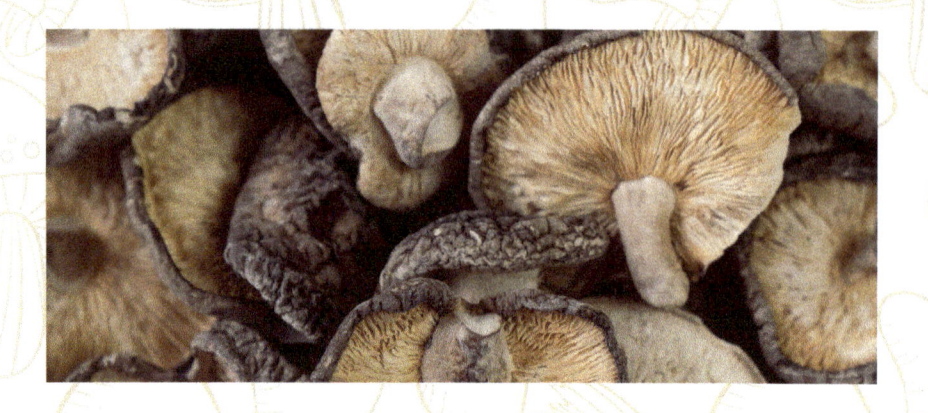

Dried Shiitake

12. Laricifomes Officinalis (Agarikon Mushroom)

The common name of this mushroom is agarikon, and it is one of the oldest known species of mushrooms. These mushrooms are relatively rare and have a unique beehive-like appearance. They are native to the regions of Europe and certain parts of northern America.

These medicinal mushrooms have two essential compounds known as agaric acid and polysaccharide. The agaric acid present in them is an anti-inflammatory compound.

These mushrooms have certain compounds that are believed to treat bacterial, viral, and fungal infections. Their antiviral and antibacterial properties help fight the common flu and other mild infections.

Even fungal infections such as e- coli and candida can be treated with these mushrooms. Since they are rich in anti-inflammatory compounds, any pain and health problems caused by inflammation such as arthritis, kidney inflammation, and lumbago can be treated with them.

They also have immune-boosting functions. Apart from all these health benefits, these mushrooms are also believed to improve and maintain the health of the gastrointestinal tract.

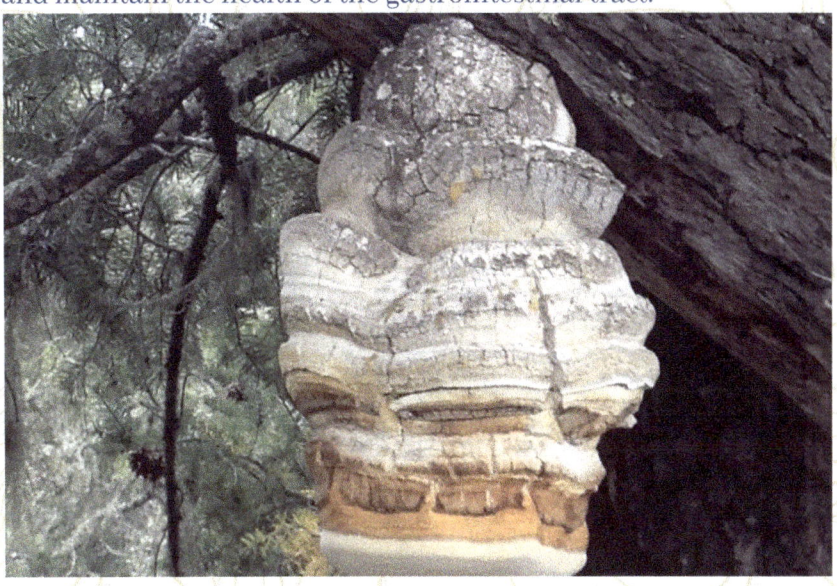

agarikon
Photo Attribution: Steph Jarvis, CC BY-SA 3.0 <https://creativecommons.org/licenses/by-sa/3.0>, via Wikimedia Commons

13. Psilocybin Cubensis (Magic Mushrooms)

Magic mushrooms are known as psilocybin cubensis and are known for their psychedelic properties. Though they were relatively obscure, they are slowly gaining popularity because of their different benefits.

These mushrooms in their dried form can cause a high or a psychedelic effect due to high levels of psilocybin. That said, with micro-dosing and careful pressing, psychiatric conditions such as anxiety, depression, and post-traumatic stress disorder can be treated with these extracts.

Magic mushrooms accelerate the formation of new brain cells and connections. They also promote neuronal regeneration. Combining these factors improves one's ability to concentrate, become more creative, and strengthen cognitive skills.

For now, it's essential to understand that these mushrooms are being considered as a potential option for treating persistent depressive disorders, cluster headaches, anxiety, substance abuse disorders, and withdrawal, along with other psychiatric applications.

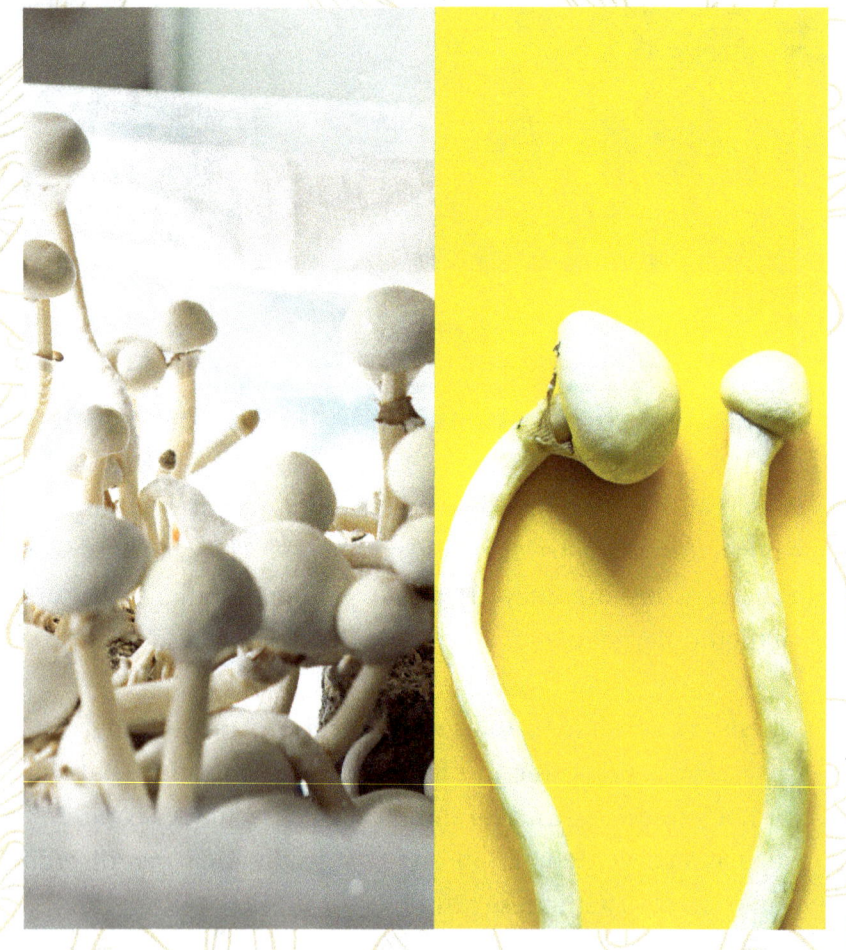

psilocybin cubensis

15. Tricholoma Matsutake (Matsutake Mushrooms)

These are commonly known as matsutake mushrooms and are found in North America, northern Europe, and East Asia.

These are some of the best-tasting edible mushrooms. These mushrooms are rather hard to find and quite expensive. They are a rich source of B complex vitamins, zinc selenium, protein, copper, and potassium.

Since they are rich in dietary fiber and other healthy minerals, they are believed to reduce cholesterol levels while stimulating better digestion and relieving constipation.

They are among the costliest mushrooms known and also have cancer-fighting properties.

From preventing the hardening of arteries to improving cardiovascular health and energy metabolism, there are a lot of benefits offered by these mushrooms.

They are also known to strengthen the bones and teeth due to high levels of vitamin D.

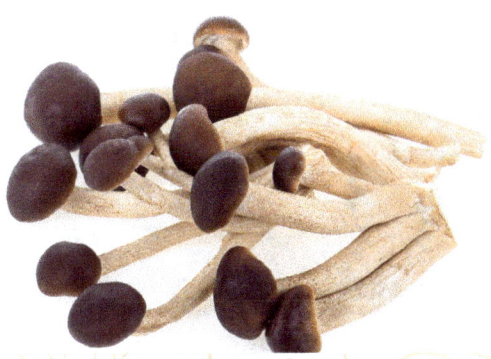

Matsutake Mushrooms

16. Calvatia Gigantea (Giat Puffballs)

These mushrooms are commonly known as giant puffballs. This is because they are incredibly delicious and have a host of medicinal properties. In addition, they are saprotrophic fungi and feed on organic matter in the wild.

Because of their large size and color, they are known as giant puffballs.

A substance known as clavacin is present in them and is believed to promote anti-tumor activities. This gives these mushrooms the ability to suppress the duplication of cancer cells and tumors in the body.

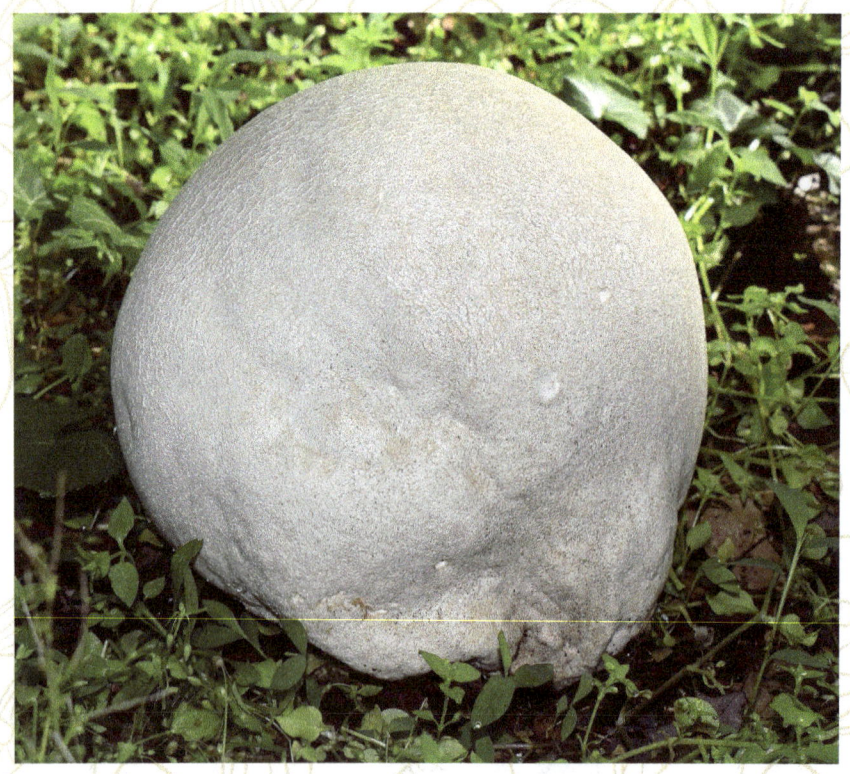

Giant Puffball

16. Hypsizygus Tessellatus (Clamshell Mushrooms)

These mushrooms are commonly known as clamshell mushrooms, beech mushrooms, or white or brown beech mushrooms.

They have a mild and earthy flavor. In the wild, they commonly grow near beech trees and hence their name. These mushrooms are rich in a variety of nutrients that strengthen the functioning of the immune system while giving your body all the nutrients it needs.

They are also low in cholesterol and prevent the formation of atherosclerotic lesions. They also prevent parasitic infections and have antifungal properties. Apart from it, they are known to tackle inflammation because they are rich in antioxidants, promote weight loss and management, and tackle diabetes by rebalancing blood sugar levels. Certain helpful compounds present in it are known as glycoproteins that suppress the formation of cancer cells and are a good source of anti-cancer agents.

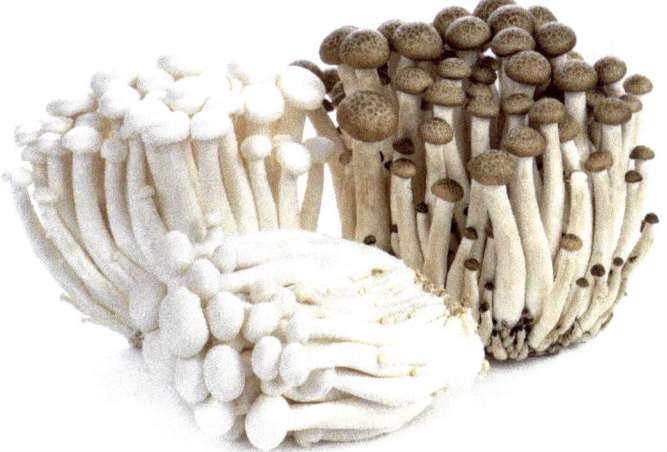

Brown & White Beech Mushrooms

17. Ophiocordyceps Sinensis

These mushrooms were previously known as Cordyceps Sinensis, and the benefits they offer are the same as those provided by Cordyceps that were discussed earlier(liver and kidney health, promoting better blood circulation, treating asthma, and reducing blood pressure levels).

These fascinating mushrooms are adaptogens and are commonly used as pre-workout supplements because of their energy-boosting abilities.

These are rather rare when compared to the cordyceps that were discussed previously. They are native to regions of Asia and are found in the wild in both China and Japan.

It is brown in color and found naturally whereas cordyceps militaris is artificially grown in labs and is yellow or white in color.

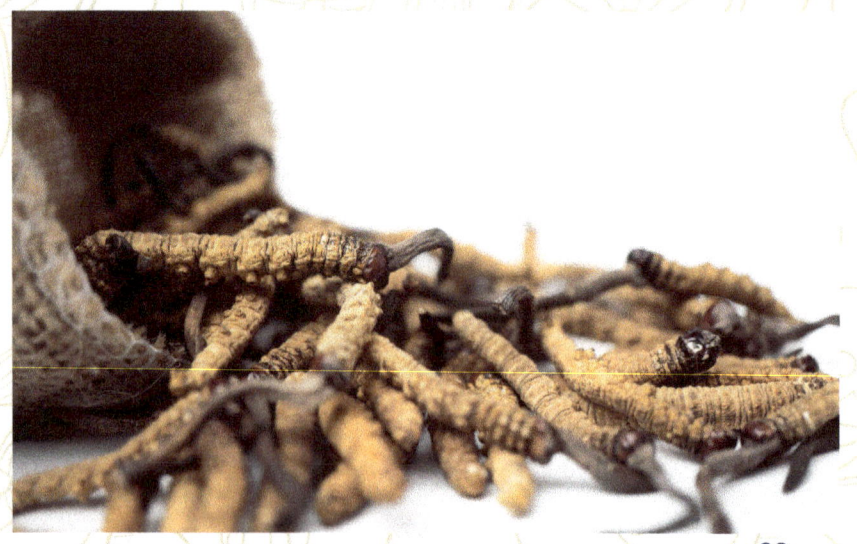

Ophiocordyceps Sinensis or Caterpillar Fungus

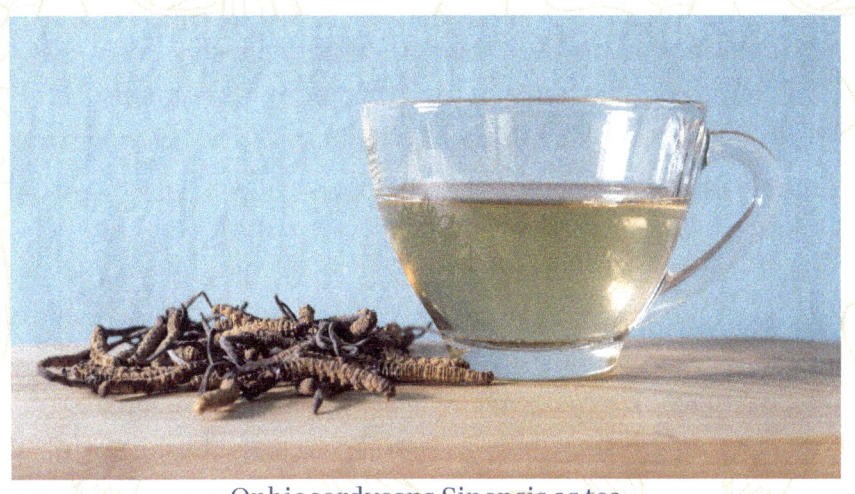

Ophiocordyceps Sinensis as tea

18. Pleurotus Ostreatus (Oyster Mushroom)

The common name of this mushroom is the oyster mushroom. However, this is not only an edible variety but is commonly used for its medicinal properties.

The natural compounds present in it are believed to help regulate the levels of blood cholesterol. This mushroom usually thrives in temperate climatic regions. These mushrooms have seven phenolic compounds but are natural antioxidants such as chlorogenic acid, gallic acid, and naringenin. They help combat oxidative stress and tackle inflammation. According to the findings of Nihad M Abdel-Monem et al. (2020), the antioxidants present in this mushroom's extracts can reduce liver damage caused by toxic chemicals present within.

They inhibit oxidative damage within the arterial cells and lower low-density lipoprotein, also known as bad cholesterol, due to ergothioneine's helpful amino acid. When LDL is oxidized, it reduces the plaque buildup in arteries resulting in a condition known as atherosclerosis. This, in turn, reduces the risk of cardiovascular disorders.

Beta-glucans are natural fibers present in this mushroom that are fermented by the gut microbiome. This automatically reduces the prediction of cholesterol in the body. According to Inga Schneider et al. (2011), consuming about 30 grams of dried extract of these mushrooms daily can reduce the levels of cholesterol and triglycerides.

Apart from this, oyster mushrooms can also reduce blood pressure and insulin levels, according to Lisa Dicks and Sabine Ellinger (2020). A combination of all these factors shows oyster mushrooms help improve cardiovascular health while reducing the risk of heart diseases.

Furthermore, the authors of the same study noticed that taking a powder of these mushrooms reduces blood sugar levels even after eating. This could be because these mushrooms promote sugar utilization in the body while reducing the effect of proteins responsible for elevating blood sugar levels.

Oyster mushrooms are believed to help promote immune functioning. For instance, the beta-glucan fibers present in them have immune-modulating properties. It is also believed to have antibacterial and antiviral properties too. Ingrid Urbancikova et al. (2020) noticed that using an oyster mushroom supplement and vitamin C and zinc can reduce the symptoms of herpes simplex virus type 1 (HSV-1).

Apart from it, it can also reduce the severity and duration of the respiratory symptoms associated with this condition. Aiko Tanaka et al. (2016) noticed that the regular use of an oyster mushroom extract supplement promotes the functioning of the immune system by strengthening its ability to fight infections.

White Oyster

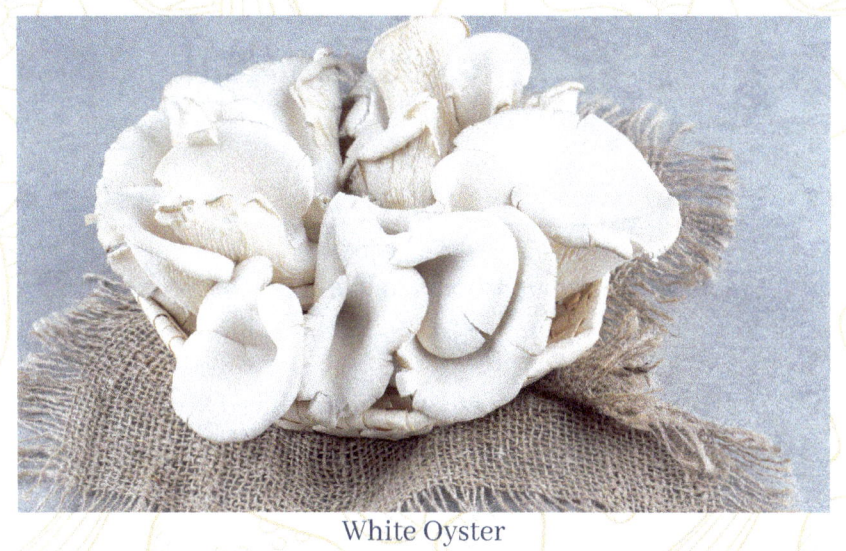

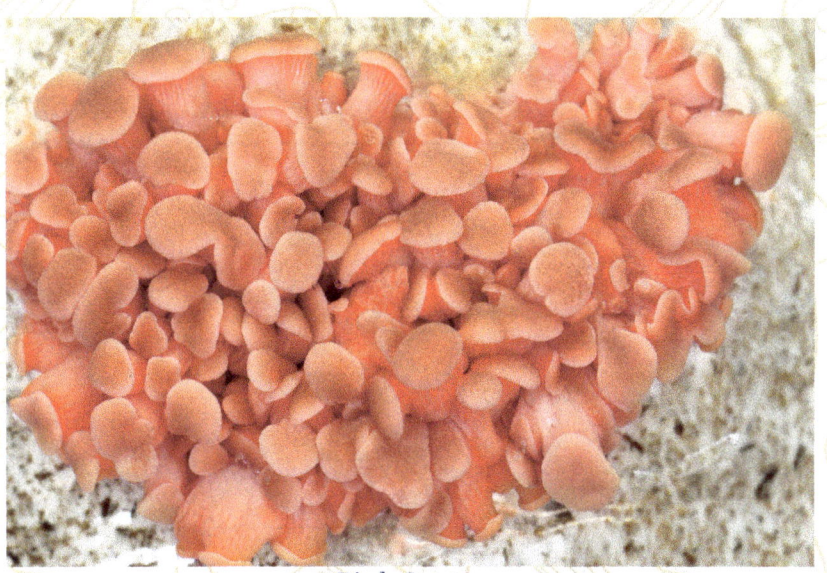

Pink Oyster

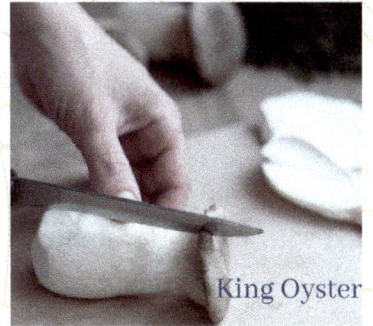

King Oyster

3. How Mushrooms Heal

A meal without mushrooms is like a day without rain.

— John Cage

In the previous chapter, you were introduced to a variety of mushrooms and all their medicinal properties. Apart from it, there are several other health conditions that mushrooms improve.

Let's look at all the different health benefits associated with mushrooms

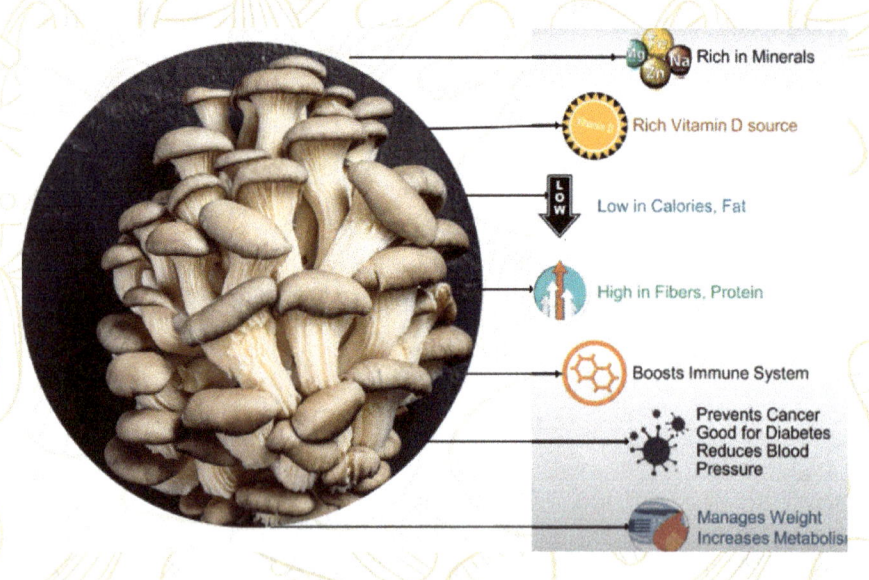

- Rich in Minerals
- Rich Vitamin D source
- Low in Calories, Fat
- High in Fibers, Protein
- Boosts Immune System
- Prevents Cancer
- Good for Diabetes
- Reduces Blood Pressure
- Manages Weight
- Increases Metabolism

Mushroom Benefits

Aging

Mushrooms are filled with helpful compounds such as vitamins, amino acids, lipids, proteins, and phenols.

They are believed to have plenty of antioxidants promoting anti-inflammatory action within the body. Topical application of different mushrooms such as tremella, shiitake, and maitake can improve skin health.

Most skin problems are caused due to inflammation that's triggered by the activity of free radicals within. The antioxidants present in mushrooms tackle inflammation that comes in handy while treating skin problems. Reduction in inflammation can also reduce bouts of skin problems such as acne breakouts. Kojic acid is a skin-lightening compound, and it is found in most mushrooms.

Unlike harmful chemicals used for skin lightening, mushrooms offer a natural remedy. The anti-inflammatory properties of mushrooms coupled with the antioxidants present in them promote the renewal of skin cells, promote brightening, and also improve elasticity.

A combination of all these factors will leave your skin feeling supple and looking healthier. The anti-aging properties of mushrooms cannot be overlooked.

The research was carried out at Pennsylvania State University Center for Plant and Mushroom Products for Health in State College.

Below are the findings:
- Few mushrooms contain not one but two types of antioxidants that have anti-aging properties.
- Out of 13 species tested, Porcini has maximum Antioxidant.
- Research is being carried out to find the correlation between consumption and mushroom and their effects on neurodegenerative diseases.

Link to the research: https://pubmed.ncbi.nlm.nih.gov/28530594/

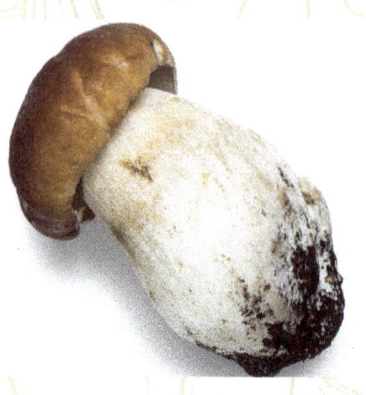

Porcini/Boletus eduli

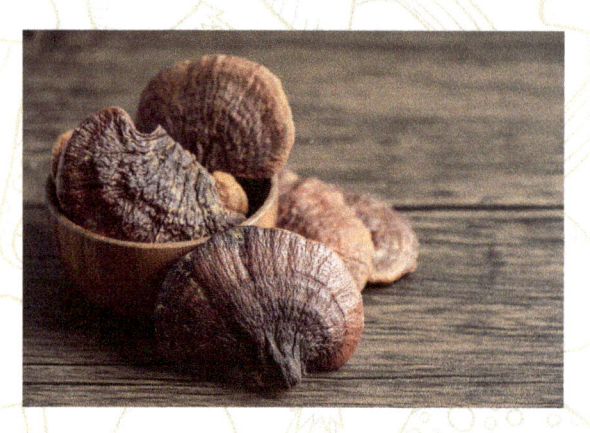

Reishi

Mushrooms with high level of antioxidants

Allergies

A practical and natural way to reduce the severity of allergy symptoms is by using a mushroom supplement, especially ones obtained from reishi and maitake mushrooms. The anti-allergic properties of reishi mushrooms reduce inflammation and promote a healthy immune system. Similarly, even maitake mushrooms can reduce the sensitivity to allergens by supporting and strengthening the function of the immune system. These mushrooms also create a natural balance within the body and promote a healthy stress response, essential for those dealing with severe allergies .

Alzheimer's

Eating mushrooms regularly can improve cognitive functioning. Those who regularly eat mushrooms can effectively reduce their risk of mild cognitive impairment or MCI. This is a precursor to degenerative disorders such as Alzheimer's. MCI causes memory troubles, problems with spatial orientation, and even language troubles.

According to Lei Feng et al. (2018), the risk of MCI reduces with regular consumption of mushrooms. The most common mushrooms associated with this reduced risk are golden, button, oyster, and shiitake mushrooms.

The authors of this study believe it is due to an antioxidant and anti-inflammatory compound known as ergothioneine (ET). The human body cannot synthesize it and its regular consumption prevents cognitive decline. The accumulation of two toxic proteins known as beta-amyloid and phosphorylated tau are associated with the onset of Alzheimer's. Natural compounds present in mushrooms can prevent their accumulation.

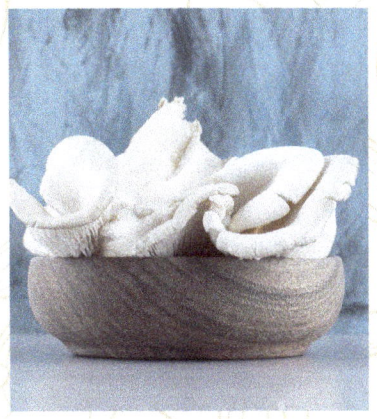

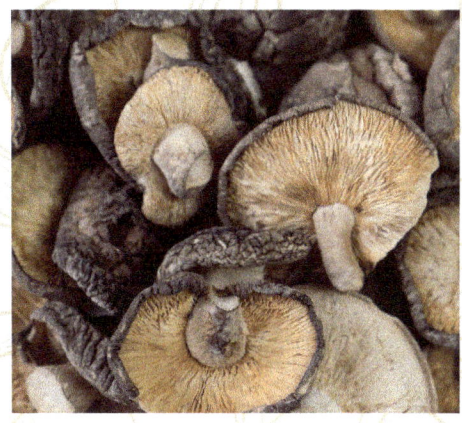

Oyster   Shiitake

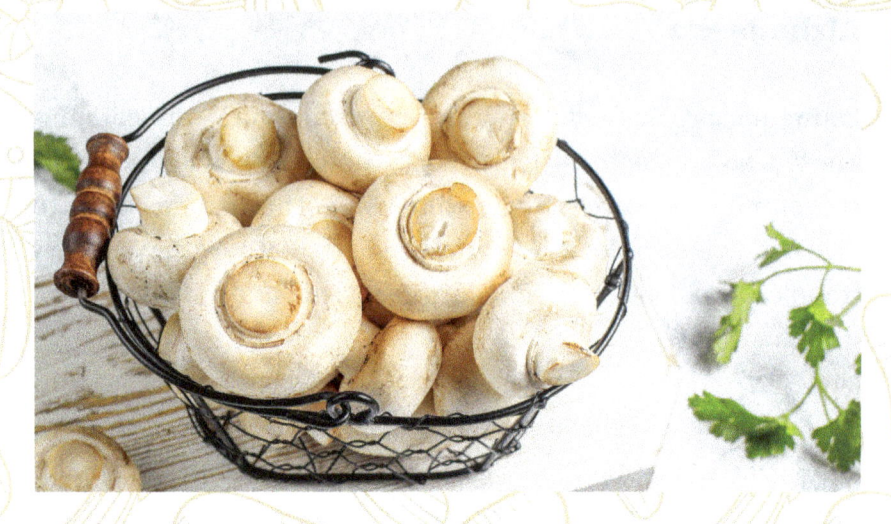

Button Mushroom

Anticoagulant

Anticoagulants are blood thinners and prevent clotting. Common examples of pharmaceutical anticoagulants include Tylenol, heparin, and aspirin. In certain medical conditions such as thrombotic disorders, blood thinners are prescribed to prevent the formation of clots. This, in turn, reduces the risk of strokes and heart attacks.

There are severe long-term side effects associated with the regular use of blood thinners. The good news is that mushrooms act as natural anticoagulants. This is associated with their antioxidant properties. Common antioxidants present in mushrooms are polysaccharides and ergosterol.

Reishi and shiitake mushrooms can reduce the risk of harmful blood clots and even slow down the process of clotting.

Cancer and Tumors

Medicinal mushrooms and extracts from them are being used as complementary dietary options for treating different types of cancer.

Mushrooms have antiviral, antibacterial, and anti-fungal properties. Apart from it, they also have certain properties that help them fight different types of cancers. Some types of mushrooms strengthen immune functioning, and this helps reduce the side effects of cancer treatment. The antioxidants present in them protect cellular DNA and reduce the damage caused by cancer-causing cells.

The beta-glucans present in them is also believed to reduce the chances of cancer relapse. They also have bioactive compounds that increase the production and longevity of white blood cells, making it easier for the body to fight the infection within. By activating an innate immune response, it accelerates different adaptive measures taken by the body to fight cancer-causing cells.

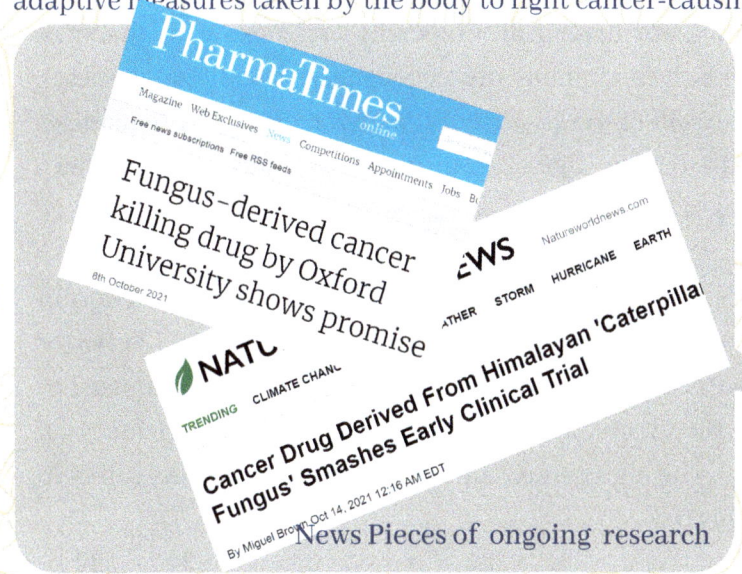

News Pieces of ongoing research

Diabetes

Diabetes means abnormally high levels of blood sugar beyond what the body can manage. Mushrooms are a few foods that can be consumed without any worries because of their high nutritional value.

Glycemic load and glycemic index are two systems used for evaluating how blood sugar levels are affected when you consume carbs. They are also used for treating chronic conditions such as diabetes.

Foods are classified into three categories according to the GI method. High GI includes food between 70- 100, medium GI is 56- 69, and low GI is 1- 55. Foods with a low glycemic index don't cause any sudden spikes in blood sugar levels. For example, one cup of mushrooms has a glycemic index of 10-15, making them low glycemic index foods. So, it controls your blood sugar levels.

Mushrooms are beneficial, especially for those with diabetes. Any food rich in vitamins protects against gestational diabetes. This is excellent news, given that over 16% of pregnancies worldwide trigger diabetes in children and their mothers, according to Jasmine F Plows et al. (2018).

In addition, vitamin B intake is associated with a reduction in the risk of diabetes. According to the findings of Kristy M Porter et al. (2019), diabetes and the use of metformin (a drug used to manage blood glucose) are associated with a deficiency of vitamin B. The high content of vitamin B in mushrooms will help reduce this risk.

Mushrooms are rich in polysaccharides, a bioactive compound that is believed to have anti-diabetic properties. According to Siwen Yang et al. (2019) and Ganesan and Baojun Xu (2019), mushrooms help increase insulin resistance making it easier for the body to deal with blood sugar levels.

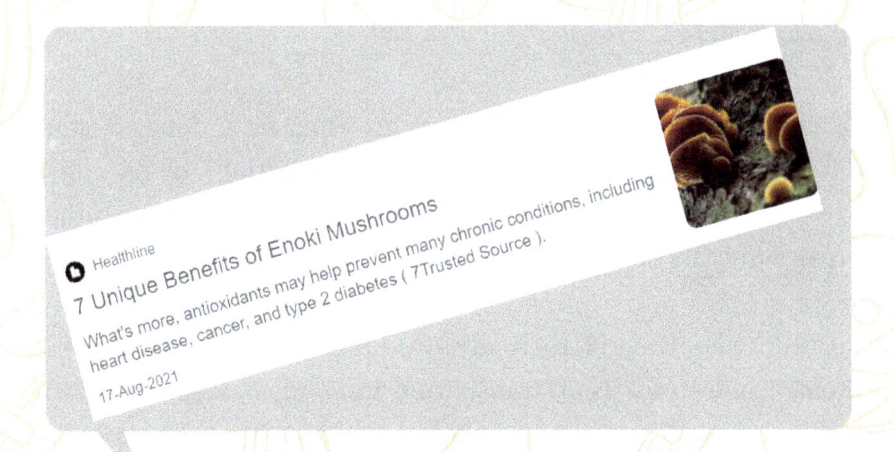

> **Healthline**
> **7 Unique Benefits of Enoki Mushrooms**
> What's more, antioxidants may help prevent many chronic conditions, including heart disease, cancer, and type 2 diabetes (7Trusted Source).
> 17-Aug-2021

Media coverage on enoki mushroom & diabetes
Link: https://www.healthline.com/nutrition/enoki-mushrooms-benefits

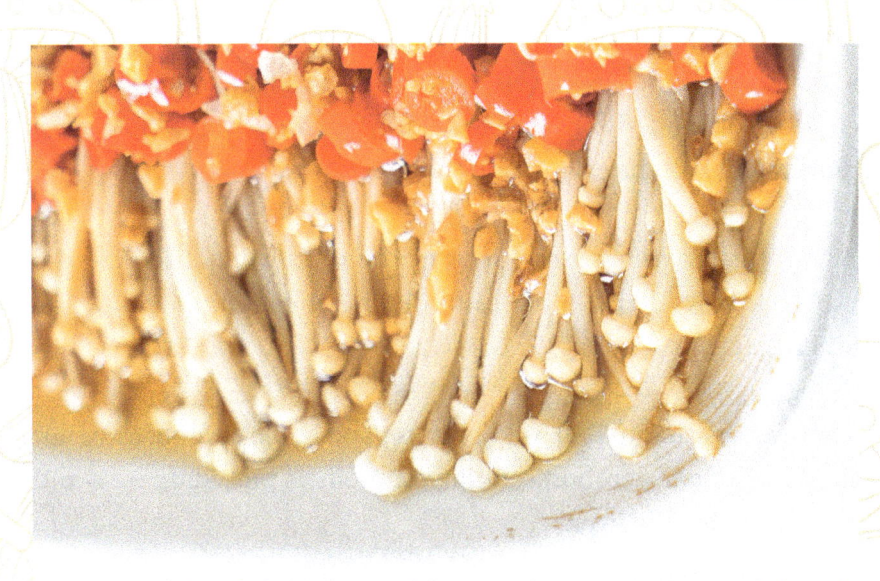

Steamed Enoki Mushroom

Cholesterol

Cholesterol essentially refers to a type of waxy substance that is commonly found in the bloodstream. Cholesterol is needed for building healthy cells. That said, excess cholesterol increases the risk of several coronary diseases, including strokes and heart attacks.

When your cholesterol levels start growing, fatty deposits start developing in the blood vessels, obstructing blood flow. Eventually, it results in a situation where these deposits either break suddenly or form clots resulting in stroke or heart attacks.

Regarding cholesterol, there are two lipoproteins responsible for them. Cholesterol is a transporter in your bloodstream is a combination of proteins and cholesterol known as a lipoprotein. Depending on what the lipoprotein carries, there are different types of cholesterol.

Usually, they're divided as low-density lipoprotein or LDL and high-density lipoprotein or HDL. LDL is also known as bad cholesterol and is responsible for transporting cholesterol molecules to all the cells in your body.

When this level increases, it causes the narrowing of the arterial walls making them hard, resulting in a condition known as atherosclerosis.

On the other hand, HDL is known as good cholesterol because all the excess cholesterol present in your body is picked up by it and transported to the liver.

The findings of Sang Chul Jeong et al. (2009) suggest that the consumption of button mushrooms or Agaricus bisporus helps reduce and regulate cholesterol and blood sugar levels in hypercholesterolemic and diabetic rats. Similar results were obtained from a study on rats conducted by Shanggong Yu et al. (2016) using shiitake mushrooms. In addition, Tanya T W Chu et al. (2012) noticed that reishi mushrooms help regulate and rebalance the cholesterol and triglyceride levels during a controlled 12-week human study.

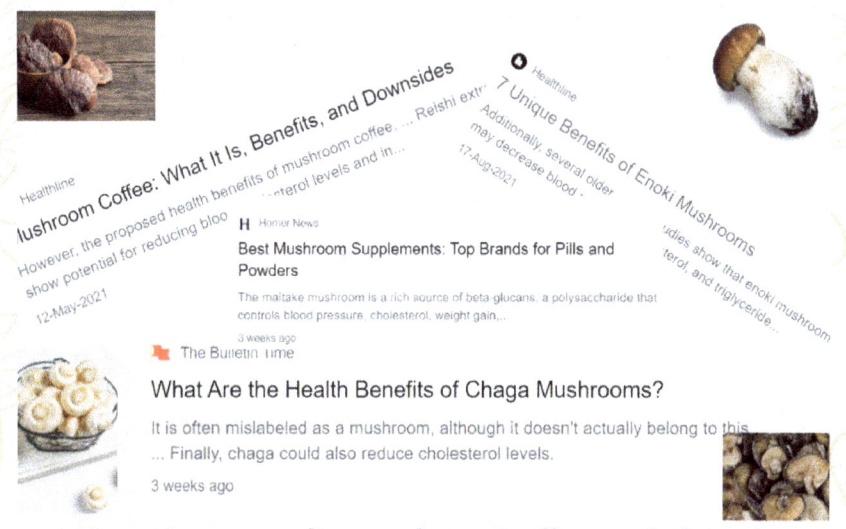

News pieces regarding mushroom's affect on cholestrol

Hearing Loss

Most of us associate vitamin D with bone health. The ear is composed of several delicate bones. Vitamin D from mushrooms helps keep these bones healthy and strong. This, in turn, can improve your ear health and indirectly reduce the risk of hearing loss.

Regulate Blood Pressure

Hypertension is a prevalent disorder these days, and it is known as high blood pressure as well. In this condition, the pressure exerted by blood on the arterial walls increases drastically, leading to health problems, including cardiovascular disorders. The amount of blood pumped by the heart and the blood flow resistance within the arteries determines the normal blood pressure. The more blood the heart pumps and the narrower the arteries become, the higher blood pressure.

According to an animal study conducted by Y Kabir and S Kimura (1989), the consumption of mushrooms helps reduce blood pressure. Certain compounds present in reishi and polypore mushrooms help reduce the effects of hypertension. Reishi helps regulate the angiotensin-converting enzyme (ACE) that is responsible for regulating blood pressure levels.

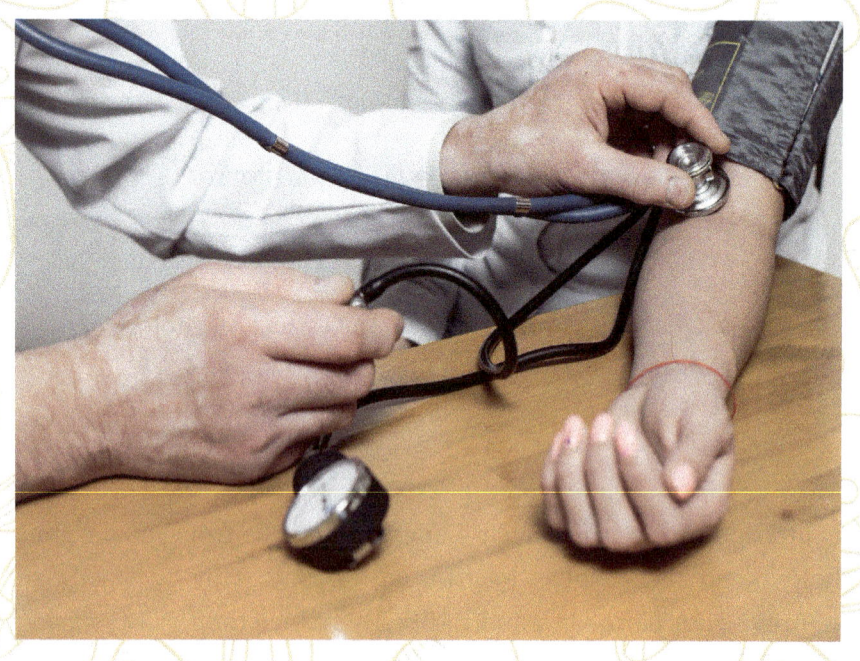

Blood Pressure Test

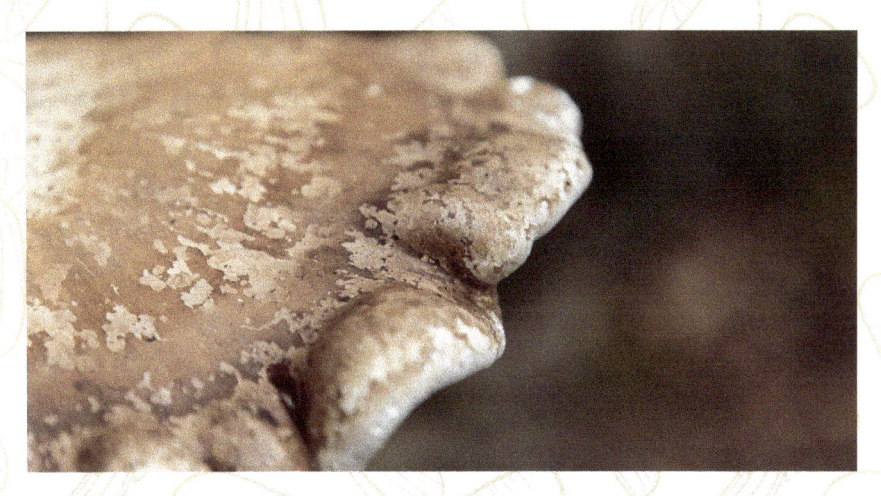

Polypore Mushroom

Immune System

Mushrooms are a great addition to your diet, especially if you want to improve the functioning of your immune system. The immune system is your body's first line of defense against infections and potential illnesses. The immune system also ensures all your internal functions and systems are working effectively and efficiently. Your body's ability to produce antibodies, T cells, B cells, macrophage, and cytokines are directly affected by mushrooms. All these are natural killer cells and play an important role in your immune system. According to the findings of M Jayachandran et al. (2017), mushrooms help strengthen the functioning of the immune system by stimulating the production of anti-inflammatory cytokines and suppressing pro-inflammatory cytokinin.

At the start of an infection, mushrooms trigger the production of inflammatory cytokines that help your body fight off the invaders. After this, they begin an anti-inflammatory response to calm down the immune system. So in this sense, mushrooms act as immune modulators.

A more robust immune system reduces the risk of infections like chronic inflammation and ensures speedy recovery. Chronic inflammation is a painful condition causing other illnesses such as rheumatoid arthritis, multiple sclerosis, neurodegenerative diseases, and cardiovascular disorders.

When the immune system isn't functioning properly, it mistakenly attacks healthy cells causing autoimmune disorders. Inflammation is the immune system's first line of defense against pathogens and other illnesses. If this is left unchecked and doesn't reduce, it causes severe health complications. The antioxidants found in mushrooms help regulate inflammation.

Bioactive compounds known as polysaccharides along with beta-glucans found in mushrooms act as biological response modifiers. They play an important role in strengthening your body's innate and adaptive immune system. If you want to improve the functioning of your immune system, start consuming turkey tail mushrooms, shiitake, maitake, chaga, reishi, and cordyceps regularly.

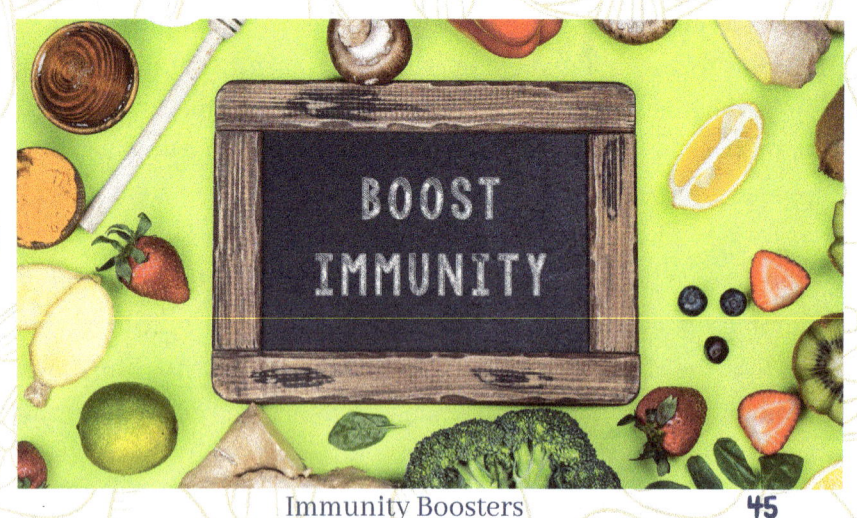

Immunity Boosters

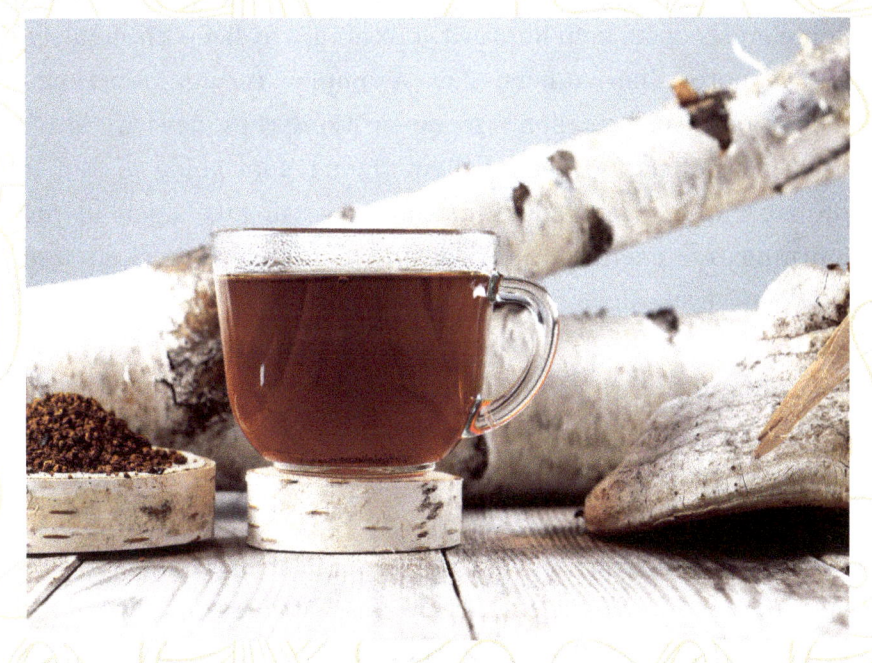

Chaga Mushroom Tea

Insomnia

Consumption of mushrooms is believed to help regulate the circadian rhythm. It is responsible for your sleep-wake cycle. Any disturbance in this rhythm makes it difficult to fall asleep at night or stay awake during the daytime. Some mushrooms help balance mental and physical stress levels, making it easier to sleep at night. They are also known to strengthen the functioning of the immune system.

For hundreds of years now, traditional Chinese medicine has used reishi mushrooms to treat insomnia and restlessness. According to the findings of Xiang-Yu Cui et al. (2012), extracts of reishi mushrooms help prolong the duration of sleeping, including the deeper state of sleep known as non-rapid eye movement (Non-REM) sleep.

Some mushrooms help improve your ability to sleep through the night more than others. For example, certain functional mushrooms such as lion's mane or Cordyceps have a rather energizing effect. So, taking them right before going to bed is probably not a good idea. Instead, you can take them in the morning to re-energize your body and mind then get acclimatized to staying awake during the day without feeling sleepy.

According to the research undertaken by Hardeep S. Tuli et al. (2014), cordyceps can improve physical stamina along with energy levels. In addition, the findings of Young Shik Park et al. (2002) suggest that Lion's mane mushrooms have the unique ability to stimulate the production of brain-derived neurotrophic factors and nerve growth factors. These are two essential proteins responsible for the normal functioning of nerve cells that keep you awake during the day.

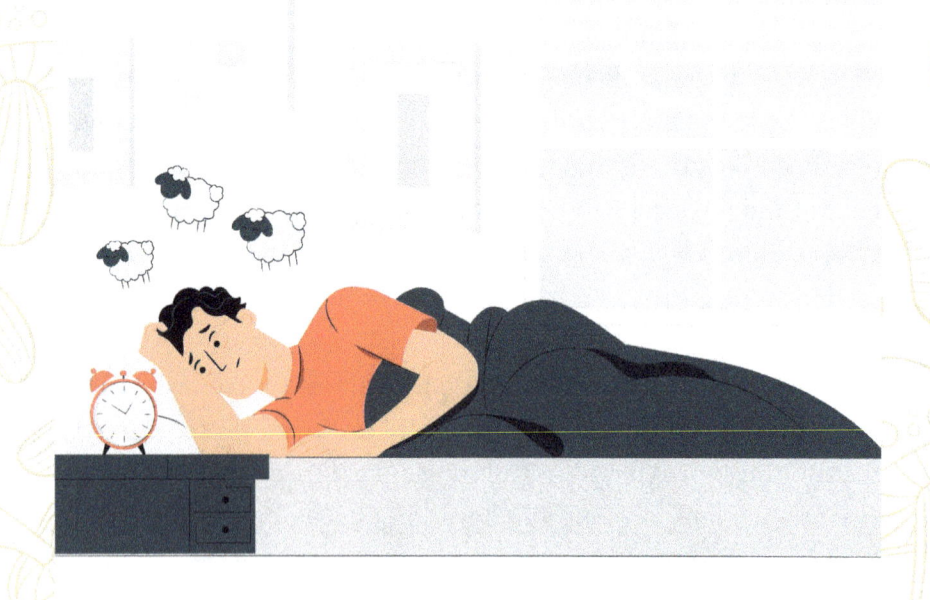

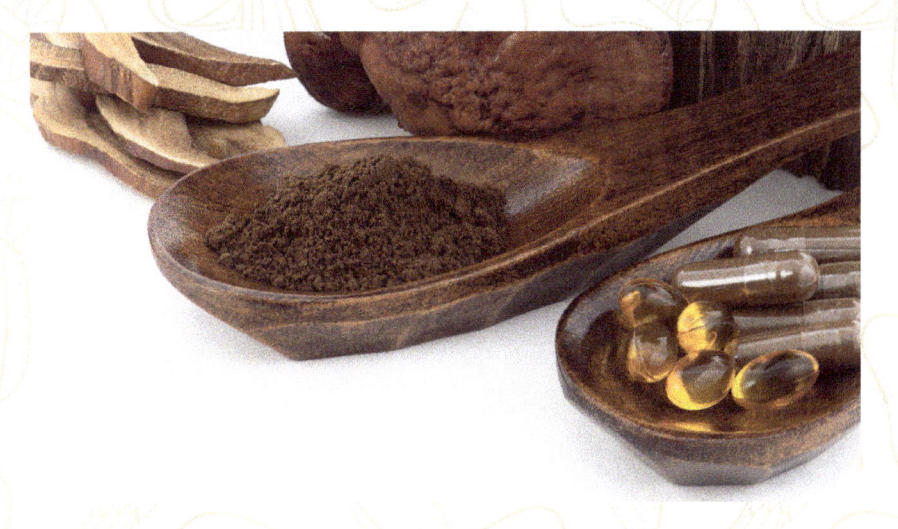

Reishi Mushroom Powder & Pills

Inflammation

Inflammation is the immune system's first response across any infections, pathogens, or foreign bodies. Inflammation is triggered whenever the immune system detects any of the pathogens mentioned above or potential infection-causing agents. Unfortunately, if this inflammation doesn't reduce even after the potential threat is eliminated, it is known as chronic inflammation. This also increases the risk of developing several harmful health problems and diseases, including cardiovascular disorders, bowel diseases, etc.

A simple way to reduce inflammation in your body is by increasing your consumption of mushrooms. There are two primary ways in which mushrooms tackle information. First, they contain anti-inflammatory compounds along with antioxidants. Second, mushrooms contain antioxidants along with fennels that provide anti-inflammatory protection in your body.

Apart from this, helpful compounds known as triterpenes are also present in mushrooms. These compounds act as natural steroids and tackle inflammation by addressing its root cause instead of simply treating the symptoms. According to Se Young Choi et al. (2010), the consumption of mushrooms promotes an anti-inflammatory response in the body. Since inflammation is associated with several other conditions such as colitis and Irritable bowel syndrome (IBS), you can reduce the risk of these diseases by reducing inflammation.

> Qrius
> **Lion's Mane Mushrooms Can Boost Health Naturally**
> Lion's mane mushrooms are loaded with anti-inflammatory compounds, ... by protecting against the growth of a bacteria called H. pylori.

News byte on Anti-Inflammatory properties of Lion's Mane Mushroom

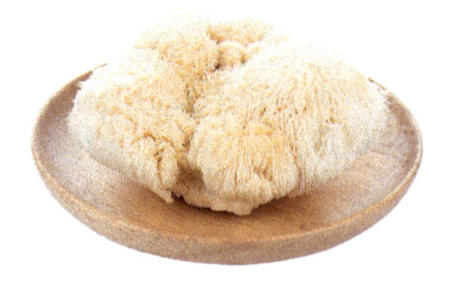

Lion's Mane

Gut Health

Mushrooms are filled with dietary fiber. This fiber comes in handy, especially if you are trying to improve your gut health.

Dietary fiber is the best prebiotic you can consume for strengthening gut functioning. Your gut is home to millions of microbes known as the gut microbiome.

These microbes need sustenance just like any other living beings, and prebiotic fibers provide this much-needed sustenance. As long as the bacteria get what they need to eat to thrive, your gut's health improves. Thus, improving your gut health automatically enhances your overall well-being as well.

For instance, any dysfunction in your gut starts showing up as skin troubles. If you want to clear your complexion or reduce the risk of skin troubles, incorporate mushrooms into your diet. The growth of helpful gut microbes such as Bifidobacterium and Lactobacillus increases when they get plenty of dietary fiber from mushrooms.

When the gut is functioning properly, the risk of developing irritable bowel syndrome also reduces. In this condition, the gut lining weakens. When this happens, undigested food can easily enter the bloodstream triggering an immune response. As mentioned, mushrooms strengthen immune functioning as well. This coupled with better gut health automatically reduces the risk of Irritable bowel syndrome (IBS) and related conditions.

Heart's Health

Improving your heart's health should be your priority, especially in times when cardiovascular diseases are steadily increasing. Whether it's coronary diseases, strokes, or heart attacks, you can reduce the risk of all this by becoming mindful of the food you consume.

Mushrooms contain fiber that is soluble and insoluble. Soluble fiber helps reduce the total level of LDL cholesterol and by cutting out this cholesterol, it automatically reduces the risk of heart diseases. Another important risk factor associated with an increased risk of heart diseases is obesity.

If you are overweight or obese, weight loss will help reduce the risk of coronary diseases. Since mushrooms are rich in dietary fiber, low in calories, and don't contain any harmful fats, it means you will feel fuller even with fewer calories. This, in turn, assists in weight loss.

Another reason how mushrooms help improve your heart health is because of the antioxidants present in them. The levels of ergothioneine, a helpful antioxidant, tackle inflammation and reduce the damage caused by oxidative stress. A combination of all these factors will automatically reduce the risk of cardiovascular disorders while improving the heart's health.

Shiitake

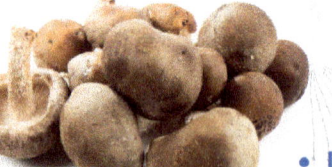

- **Lower Choestrol**
- **Improves Heart Health**
- **Improves Blood Circulation**
- **Helps in keeping optimum Blood Pressure**

Kidney Function

The kidneys are responsible for maintaining fluid balance in the body. Apart from this, they also act as the body's natural toxin elimination system. If the kidneys cannot do this, it increases swelling in the body parts. So when you start adding mushrooms to your diet, the health of your kidneys improves.

For instance, mushrooms help reduce the swelling associated with excess fluid buildup due to the inability of kidneys to maintain the ideal fluid level inside. It can also increase urine production, helping your body get rid of the accumulated toxins present within. As mentioned, mushrooms have certain helpful compounds in them responsible for reducing blood pressure or hypertension.

Hypertension is one of the risk factors associated with kidney troubles. By eliminating the risk factor itself, the chance of kidney-related issues is also reduced. Another risk factor associated with an increased risk of kidney troubles is high cholesterol. Mushrooms reduce and regulate cholesterol levels, making it easier for the kidneys to do their job effectively and efficiently.

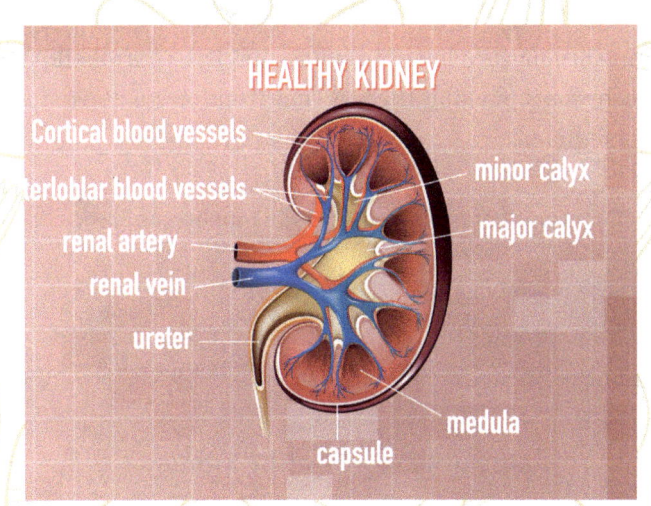

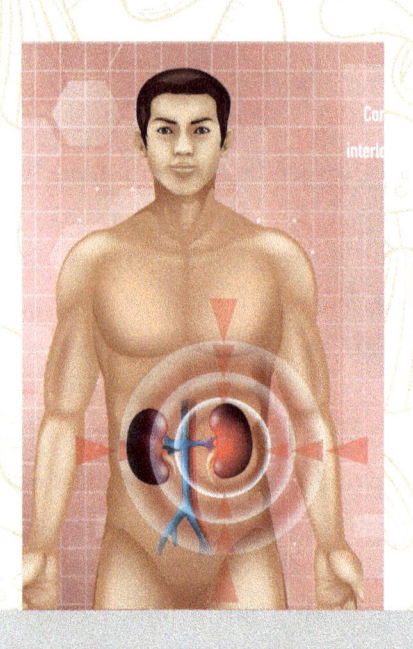

Shiitake mushrooms are a savory active ingredient that can be used as a plant-based meat replacement for those on a renal diet who need to restrict protein.

They are an outstanding resource of vitamin B, copper, manganese, and selenium.

On top of that, they provide a good quantity of plant-based protein as well as dietary fiber.

Shiitake mushrooms are lower in potassium than portobello and white switch mushrooms, making them a smart option for those following a kidney diet regimen.

One mug (150 grams) of prepared shiitake mushroom has :

- salt: 7 mg.
- potassium: 160 mg.
- phosphorus: 40 mg.

Obesity

Mushrooms are rich in protein and fiber. Combining these makes them one of the healthiest foods available, especially if you want to lose weight. They help improve your body's ability to burn fats and regulate blood sugar levels.

This, coupled with all the nutrients present in them, will improve your endurance. Mushrooms have higher nutrient density and are energizing foods without increasing your calorie intake.

A combination of this ensures you can lose weight and fat without depriving yourself of food. For instance, a cup of white mushrooms has only 15 calories while that of portobello mushrooms has 35 calories. Whenever you cook mushrooms, the volume increases, but they are still relatively low in calories when compared to all other foods.

Regarding weight loss and maintenance, an important aspect you need to concentrate on is not just the number of calories you consume but also the volume.

The volume of food you consume influences your satiety level. By opting for foods that are low in energy density, you can still eat fewer calories without feeling hungry between meals.

According to the findings of Kavita H Poddar et al. (2013), replacing red meats with mushrooms has a positive effect on overall body weight and composition. This also reduces calorie intake while promoting weight loss.

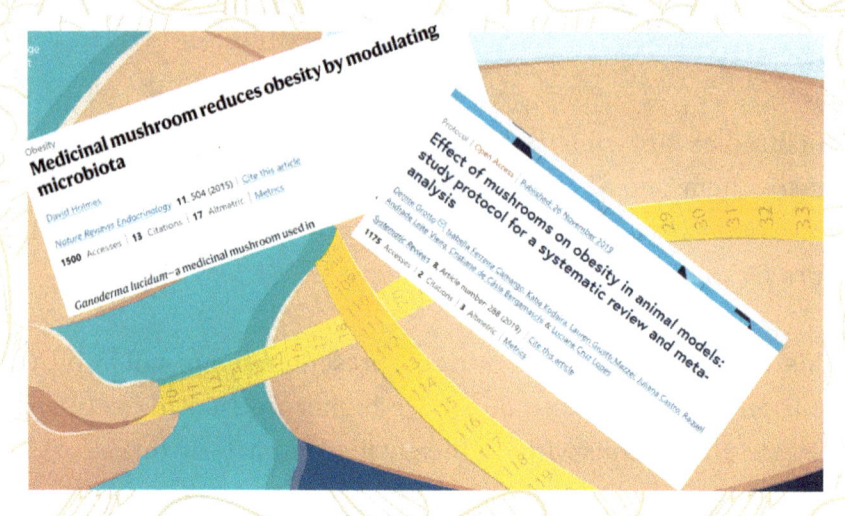

Various Research News on Mushrooms & Obesity

Mental Health

Millions of people suffer from different mental health conditions across the world. Whether it is stress, anxiety, depression, or any other disorder, they take a toll on your overall well-being. There is a connection between your mental and physical health. One cannot be optimized without the other. Simple lifestyle changes such as consuming a well-balanced diet, regulating stress levels, exercising regularly, and getting sufficient sleep will improve your mental health.

Until now, you were introduced to all the different physical health benefits of adding mushrooms to your diet. Once your physical health improves, your mental health also automatically improves. That said, an underlying medical health condition might also be the reason for the physical symptoms you are suffering from.

There are three amazing mushrooms associated with better mental health: lion's mane, reishi, and cordyceps.

Each of these mushrooms helps improve your mental health in one way or the other.

For instance, one of the most common foods associated with improving cognitive functioning and reducing the risk of neurological disorders is the lion's mane. It's believed to support and restore the nervous system. In addition, it has a calming effect that comes in handy to treat conditions such as anxiety and depression, according to Mayumi Nagano et al. (2010).

A common condition associated with mental illnesses is inflammation. By reducing the risk of inflammation, your mental health also improves. You have already been introduced to the benefits mushrooms offer when tackling inflammation and increasing the antioxidants present within. The findings of Wei Yao et al. (2015) believe the anti-inflammatory properties of lion's mane mushrooms tackle depression.

Reishi is said to have a calming effect on the mind, promoting better sleep while reducing stress. This also has several anti-inflammatory properties. The triterpenes present in it are believed to be a common compound promoting better relaxation. It is also an adaptogen that helps restore balance within your body. Reishi mushrooms support the functioning of the adrenal glands while improving resilience to stress.

The triterpenes and polysaccharide compounds found in this mushroom can help reduce anxiety and depression while improving cognitive functioning.

Cordyceps is another type of mushroom that offers neuroprotective effects. It's been commonly used in folk or traditional medicine across different cultures in Asia.

It also has strong anti-inflammatory properties that are believed to improve your body's stress response. As mentioned, the link between brain health, depression, inflammation, anxiety along other health problems cannot be overlooked. As with reishi, even cordyceps are adept at improving your ability to withstand stress

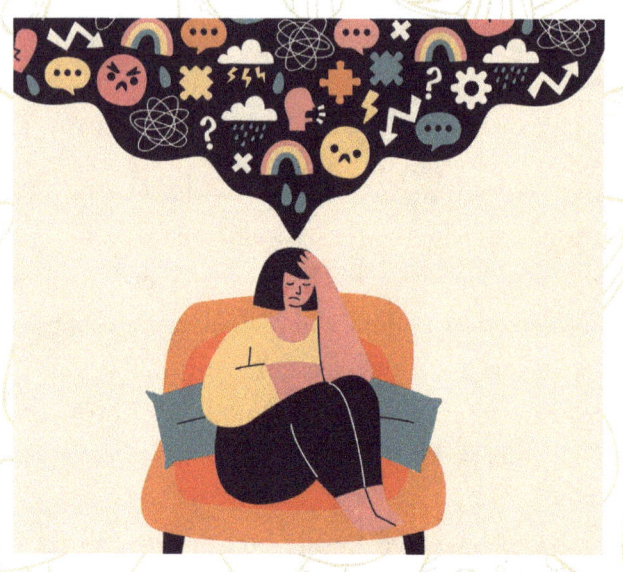

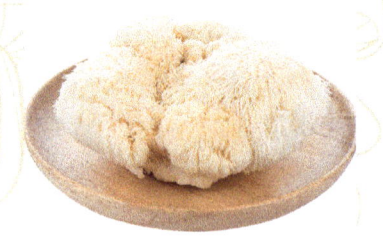

Lion's Mane

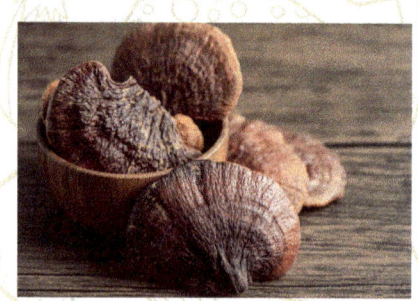

Reishi

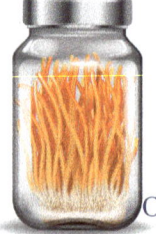

Cordyceps

Mental Health & Mushroom

Urinary Tract Infections (UTI)

Urinary tract infections or UTIs can be debilitating, mainly when they occur frequently. Millions across the world suffer from UTIs every year. When the bacterium infects the urinary tract, it causes an infection with painful and unpleasant symptoms. The usual course of treatment includes prescription antibiotics. But, as with any other pharmaceuticals, using them for too long or too frequently causes a variety of other problems as well. The good news is by focusing on your nutrition; you can reduce their occurrence. Increasing your intake of vitamin C helps.

Foods with diuretic effects such as the umbrella polypore mushroom can reduce the risk of UTIs. Even reishi mushrooms are believed to help relieve the symptoms of urinary tract infections.

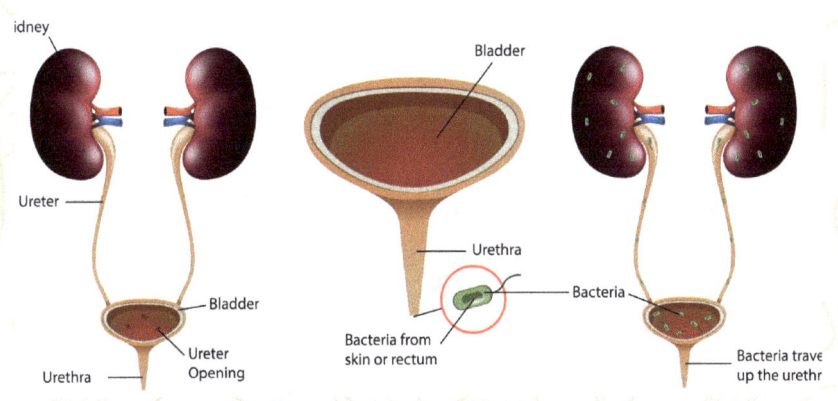

Urinary Tract Infections

Polypore Mushroom

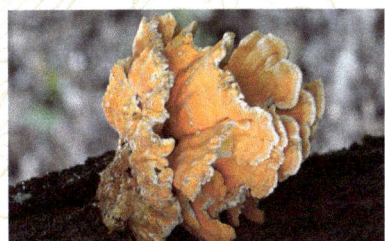

Healing

When you put all the benefits offered by mushrooms discussed in this section together, it becomes pretty clear that mushrooms promote overall healing and wellness. You can improve your overall well-being by adding mushrooms to your diet, from physical to mental health. It's essential to add a variety of mushrooms and not just restrict it to a species.

NOTE:

Before you start using any mushrooms, especially if you have pre-existing medical conditions or health problems, it's essential to consult your healthcare provider. Also, mushrooms should be used as a supplement and not adjust the soul treatment. This is important for not just your physical health but mental health as well.

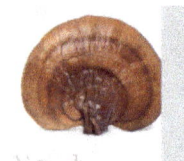

Reishi	Good Sleep, Anti-Anxiety & Depression, Increases Focus	**Chaga**	Lowering bad cholesterol, Slowing Aging, Anti-Inflammation
Lion's Mane	Increases Focus & Memory, Anti-Inflammation	**Turkey Tail**	Lowering bad cholesterol, Slowing Aging, Anti-Inflammation

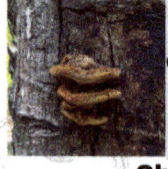

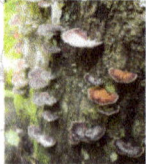

Benefits of various mushrooms

4. Identifying/Foraging Top 7 Medicinal Mushrooms

I am a mushroom
on whom the dew of heaven drops now and then."
— John Ford, The Broken Heart

1. Chaga Mushroom: The King of Medicinal Mushrooms

Chaga is just one of the most renowned fungi that are considered to have beneficial medicinal effects. If you stumble upon a birch tree, you stand a likelihood of locating Chaga, as it is generally found on both white as well as yellow birch trees.

While Chaga comes from the same fungus family, it has a distinct look. Instead, it is a parasitic development and also happens mainly on the trunks of birch trees.

You may assume it rots if you see it since they appear like a burnt blister on a birch tree.

Chaga globs tend to have a coal-black outside crust that is weak. Yet, the interior is golden brown and is often referred to as cork-like.

Suppose you're still having a hard time being able to determine the differences between *Chaga and also the Black Knot Fungus* or any other tree mushroom. In that case, that simply chip a small item of the external worlds of the mushroom with a hatchet or stone to see if that famous gold, yellow, the orange shade exists.

You intend to gather Chaga Mushrooms ethically & sustainably, so just take a tiny piece from off the mushroom's external sides and be specific to leave the tree entirely covered by the mushroom to protect from viruses.

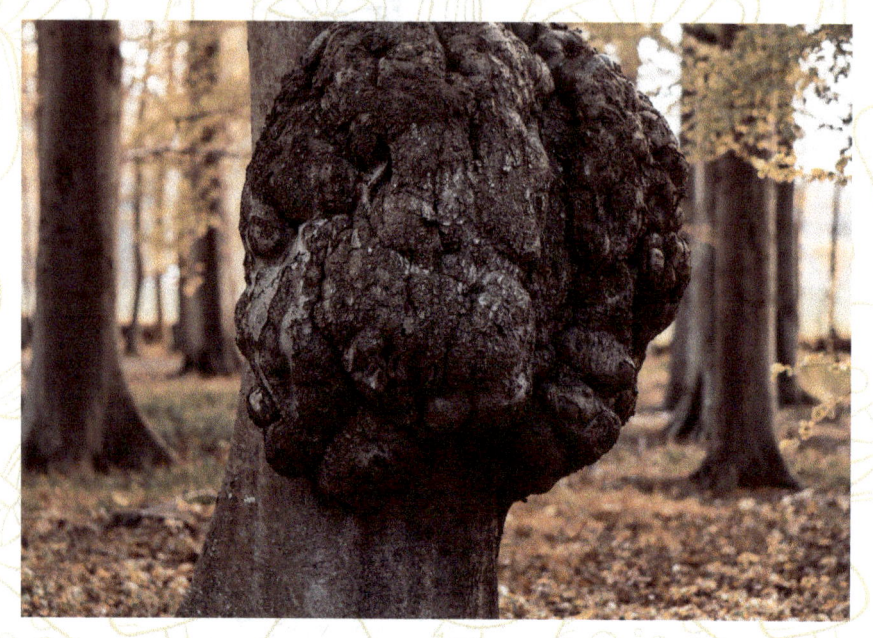

Black Knot Fungus

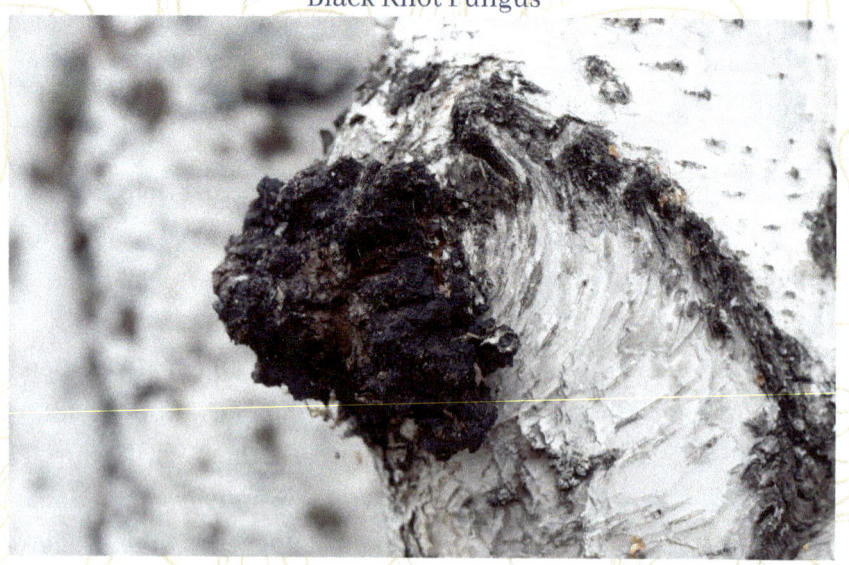

Chaga Mushroom

Burls can resemble Chaga to the untrained eye; nevertheless, Chaga has specific attributes that identify it from burls. The outward look and appearance of Chaga are blackened, charred, and hard, but it has a softer appearance and gold or brownish-yellow tone inside.

The soft amber-colored inside is the most apparent difference between chaga as well as a burl. If the growth is on something other than a birch tree, there's a likelihood that it's not chaga.

Chaga can be discovered across the northern hemisphere in locations that experience extremely cold weather. Though the majority of bountiful in Russia, North Europe, Canada as well as Alaska, a considerable quantity of Chaga can be located in the northern states of the continental united state

If you plan to harvest wild Chaga mushroom, come prepared with a sharp, saw-like blade as well as a little bit of arm muscle. The outside of Chaga is hard, and the inside is soft with golden color

Chaga identification pointers:
- You chose your mushroom from a birch tree in the northern weather area
- You located something that is charcoal-black on the tree.
- The inside is orange-yellow. It ought to seem like a cork.

After collection steps: Cleaning & Storing

- When you have collected Chaga, the next step is to break up and completely dry them.
- Begin with wiping off your fresh Chaga. See to it that there is no debris or pests in them.

- Breaking the Chaga into tiny portions, a quarter-inch across. This needs to be done promptly, as your Chaga will undoubtedly be as hard as a rock 24 hours after foraging it.
- Breaking them right into chunks will undoubtedly speed up the drying procedure and even prevent mold from expanding. It will be less complicated to make Chaga tea.
- After breaking the Chaga down, drying out will take around a month.
- As soon as dried out, you may consider grinding them to powder.

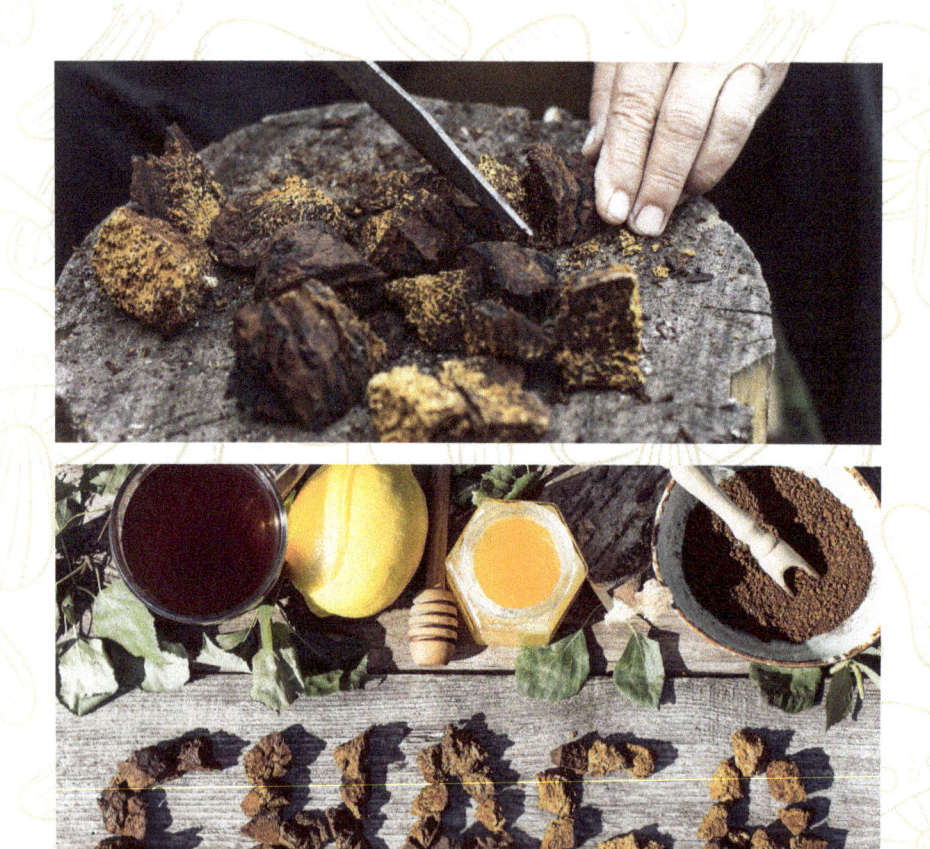

2. Reishi Mushroom: Mushroom of Immortality

Reishi or Ganoderma mushrooms pass many different names. In Asia, they're recognized by lingzhi and the mushroom of immortality. In North America, they're called varnish shelf mushrooms, artist's conk, or bear bread.

There are about 80 types of reishi mushrooms on the planet. All are shelf or brace fungi that expand on trees. Other regions will have different sorts of reishi mushrooms that look a bit different.

All reishi species grow on trees that are dead or dying. Therefore, the mushrooms will proceed to grow annually up until the timber has completely decomposed away.

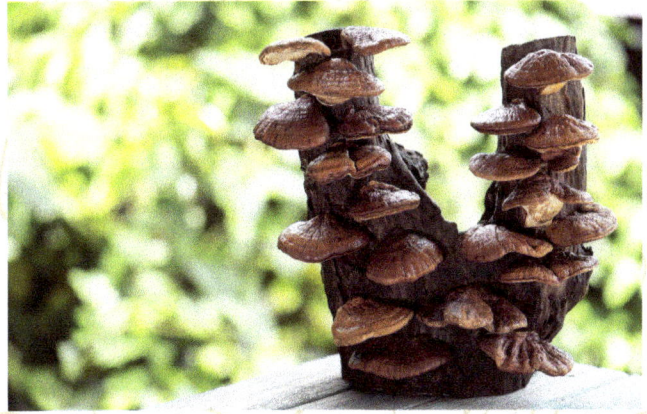

Reishi can be simple to recognize because they often have a unique look rather. For example, if you see a shelf mushroom with a deep red body as well as shades that lighten to orange, yellow, and white toward the edges of the cap, you can be sure that you're considering a reishi mushroom.

Reishi mushrooms are a kind of shelf mushroom that you can discover expanding horizontally out of the trunks of trees. They do not have any prominent stem-like mushrooms that grow out of the ground.

Older specimens might fade to a brown shade as well as be tougher to recognize. However, their scallop-shaped cap with tree-like rings on the top is a good indication.

There aren't any toxic mushrooms that look comparable to reishi mushrooms, so they're good for even newbies to attempt as well as collect. The worst-case scenario is that you'll wind up with a similar-looking mushroom that provides a great deal of extra fiber to your diet regimen; however, no real medical advantages.

Harvesting:

Make certain that the pore surface on the underside is white, ensuring that the mushroom is a young sampling. Reishi can either be carefully drawn from the tree host or chopped with a knife in softer samplings. Reishi grows at the base of trees near the ground and frequently grows around plants located growing nearby. Make certain that the mushroom you harvest hasn't grown around any hazardous plants, particularly poison ivy, which can occasionally be discovered nearby.

Storing:

Reishi mushrooms can get ruined swiftly after harvest unless they're immediately dried.

You can keep it in a paper bag stored in the fridge for 3-5 days, but the best way is when they're immediately cut into thin strips as well as dried.

Dried-out reishi mushrooms need to be stored in an impermeable container out of direct sunshine.

They can also be chopped and also made right into a reishi mushroom tincture straight after harvest, no drying required.

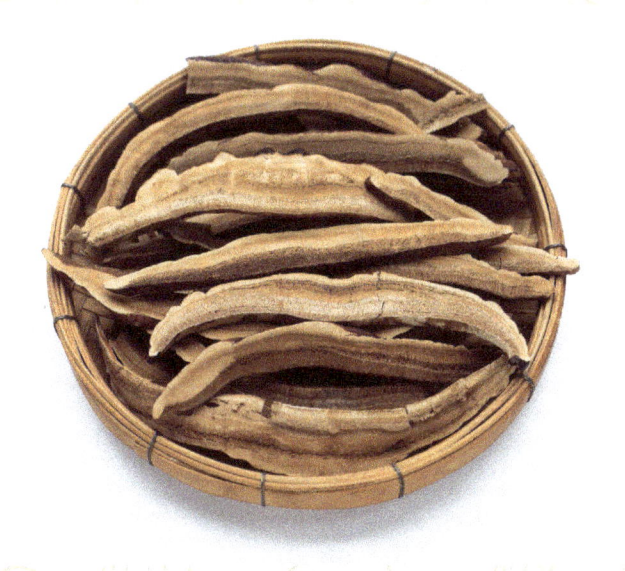

Dried Reishi

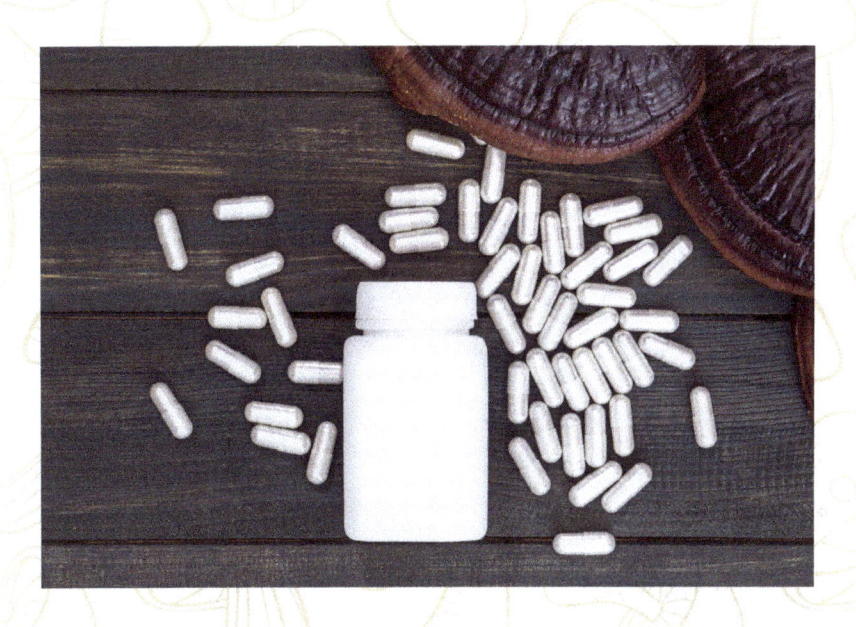

Reishi Capsules

3. Lion's Mane Mushroom

Lion's Mane Mushrooms (Hericium Erinaceus) has both culinary and medicinal value.

As soon as you find a cluster of icicles hanging from a dead hardwood, you know that it's Lion's Mane.

As an edible mushroom, lion's mane has a mild seafood taste, a little bit similar to lobster. They absorb flavors like a sponge, which makes them fit for food preparation. While they're tasty to eat, their actual worth originates from their medicinal characteristics.

What makes these mushrooms easy to recognize is that they are toothed fungi. This mushroom is a meaty, globe-shaped mushroom with cascading spinal columns. You can locate this mushroom in the spring, but you'll have even more luck finding it in the fall. There are a few hardwood trees to find this mushroom: maple, beech, oak, birch, and walnut.

The long dangling spines are unique; mushrooms in the genus Hericium have various spines; Hericium Erinaceus can be determined by spinal columns longer than 1 centimeter in length.

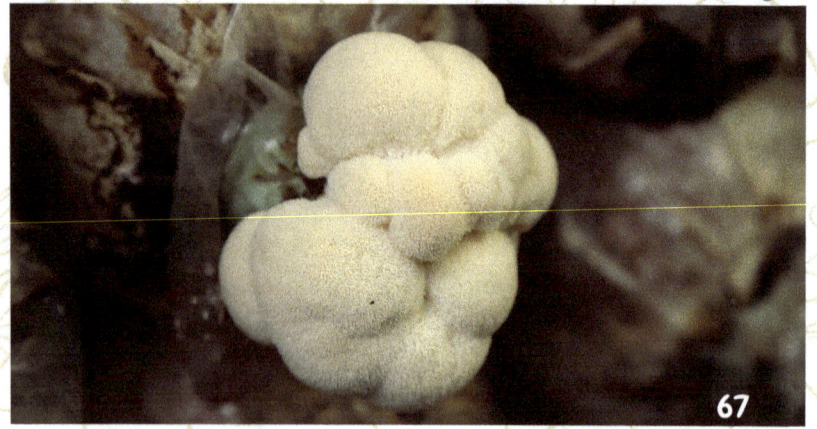

Lion's mane mushrooms are found higher up on the tree.

If you have a lot of beech trees about, along with other host trees, you can find them easily in the cold weather.

The trick is to wait for excellent weather conditions, as well as look up the tree.

If you open a mature lion's mane mushroom, you'll discover that there's little body to speak of and also a big cluster of icicle-like mushroom teeth.

Regardless of the species, they're generally white in the shade, in some cases touched with yellow or pink. Some specimens begin with a pink tinge to grow to a whiter color. As the mushrooms age, they'll yellow and also tarnish until they're a discolored orange when they mature.

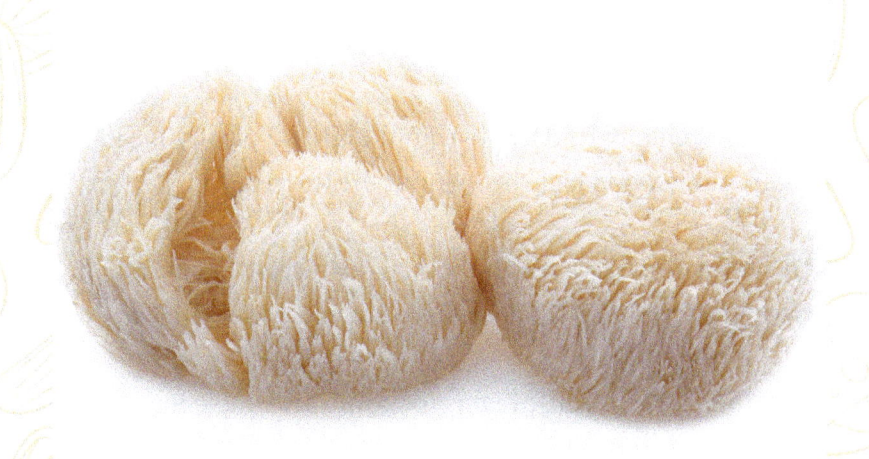

icicle-like mushroom teeth

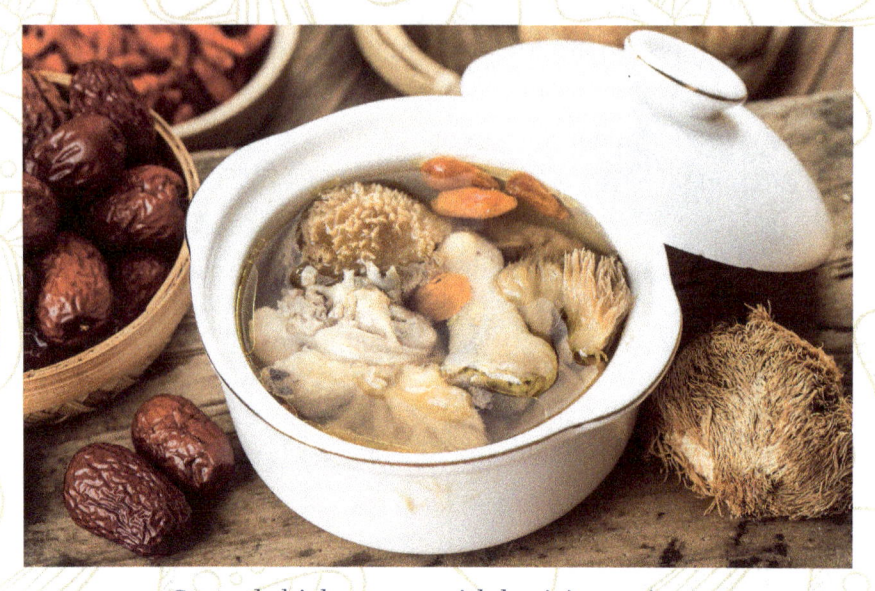

Stewed chicken soup with hericium erinaceus

4. Turkey Tail Mushroom

The stunning concentric rings of shades existing in this mushroom dependably define its scientific name: Trametes Versicolor.

Not only are Turkey Tail mushrooms aesthetically pleasing, but also easy to find!

This mushroom expands year-round and is typically located on decomposable wood logs throughout the woods.

The only tricky part about Turkey Tail mushrooms might be correctly determining them as there are many look-alikes.

Under the Turkey Tail mushroom, and also look for the tiny pores. Turkey Tail mushrooms ought to have pores on the bottom; if the underside is smooth, these mushrooms may be "false Turkey Tails" or Stereum ostrae, a sort of crust fungus.

Take a closer look. How large are the pores?

The pores in Turkey Tail are tiny that is around 4-9 pores per millimeter.

For dimension, a great trick would certainly be to make use of a ballpoint pen. Place the pen next to the pores with the pointer encountering up. The pen tip should cover at least 3+ pores. If it covers less than 3 points, the mushroom may be a different variety. If it does, you're likely to have found yourself a Turkey Tail!

Touch the surface of the mushroom. It should feel a little fuzzy, similar to the structure of velvet.

Real Turkey Tail mushrooms should also be thin and flexible, which can also inform you exactly how fresh they are; as mushrooms age, they become tough and rigid. If the mushroom you're checking out is tough or stiff, then it might be an additional type such as Trametes ochracea.

Observe the caps of the mushroom. Are there rings of varying color? If so, the colors ought to be starkly contrasting and distinctive in between one another to suggest a real turkey tail.

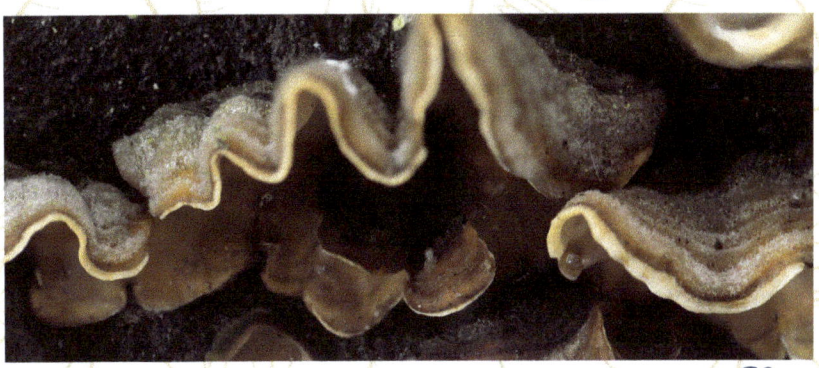

False Turkey Tail

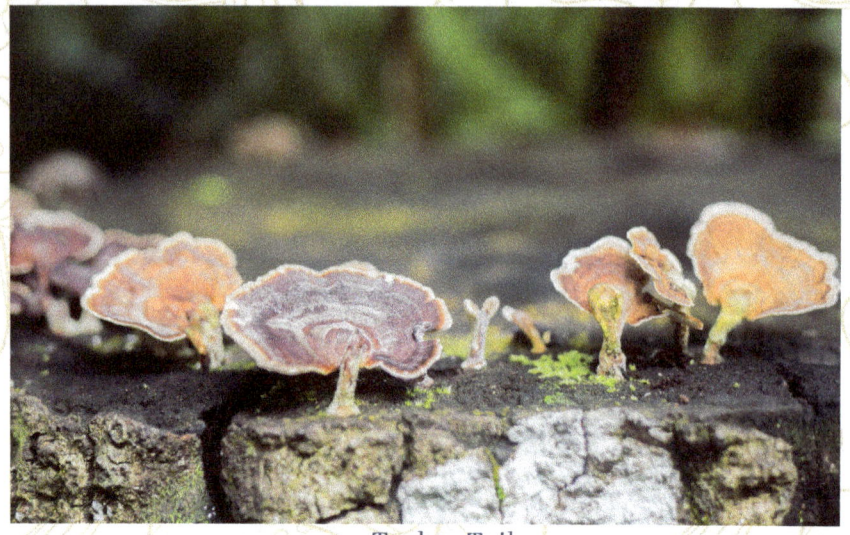

Turkey Tail

5. Cordyceps Mushroom: The Caterpillar Fungus

Cordyceps is a family of parasitic fungus that expands on the larvae of insects.

When these fungi strike their host, they replace its tissue and grow long, slender stems that expand outside the host's body.

The remains of the pest and fungi have been hand-collected, dried, and used in Chinese medicine for centuries to deal with fatigue, health issues, kidney disease, and reduced libido.

Supplements and products consisting of Cordyceps extract have ended up being significantly prominent because of their numerous supposed wellness benefits.

Out of 400 species of Cordyceps found, two have become the emphasis of wellness study: Cordyceps Sinensis and Cordyceps militaris.

Sinesis

Sinensis contains two components, stroma, and stripe.

The stroma is the upper fungal component and is dark brown or black, but can be a yellow color when new and longer than the caterpillar itself, usually 4-- 10 cm.

The stipe is slim, glabrous, and also longitudinally furrowed or jagged. It is generally found in the meadows above 3,500 meters (11,483 feet) on the Tibetan Plateau in Southwest China and the Himalayan regions of Bhutan and Nepal.

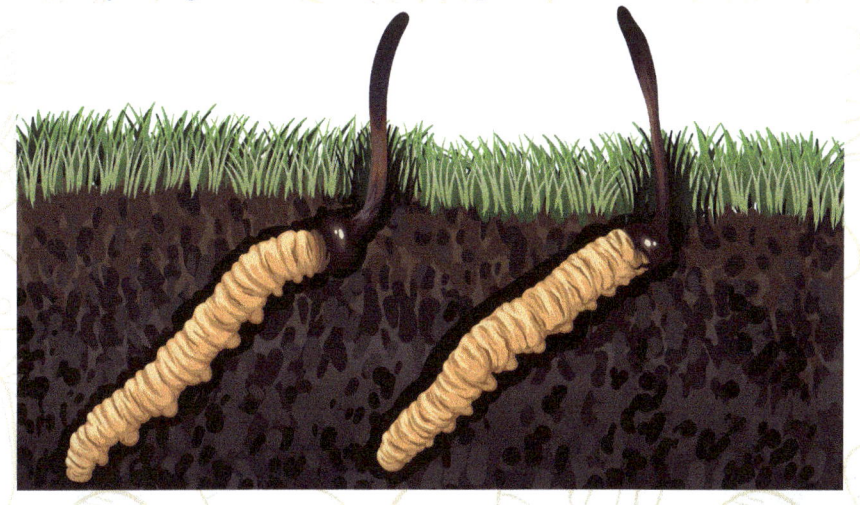

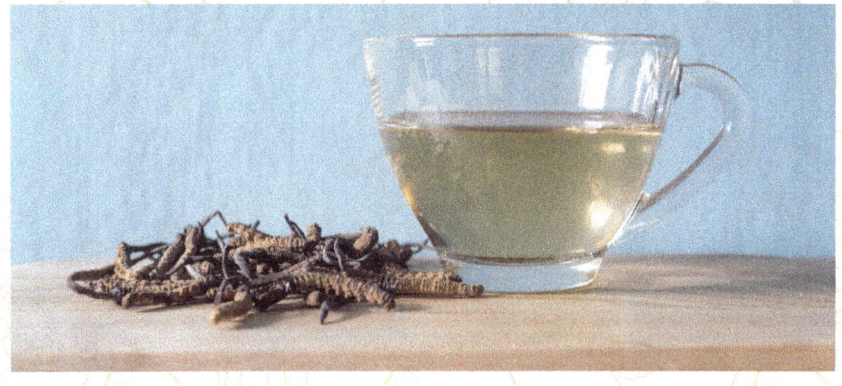

Cordyceps Sinensis

Militaris

It is like a parasite on hidden larvae and also pupae of insects (mainly moths and also butterflies).

It grows about 2-8 centimeters and is club-shaped, with the upper part wider than the base. The upper part is orange ib color.

They are naturally found in Sa - Lao Cai, Vietnam.

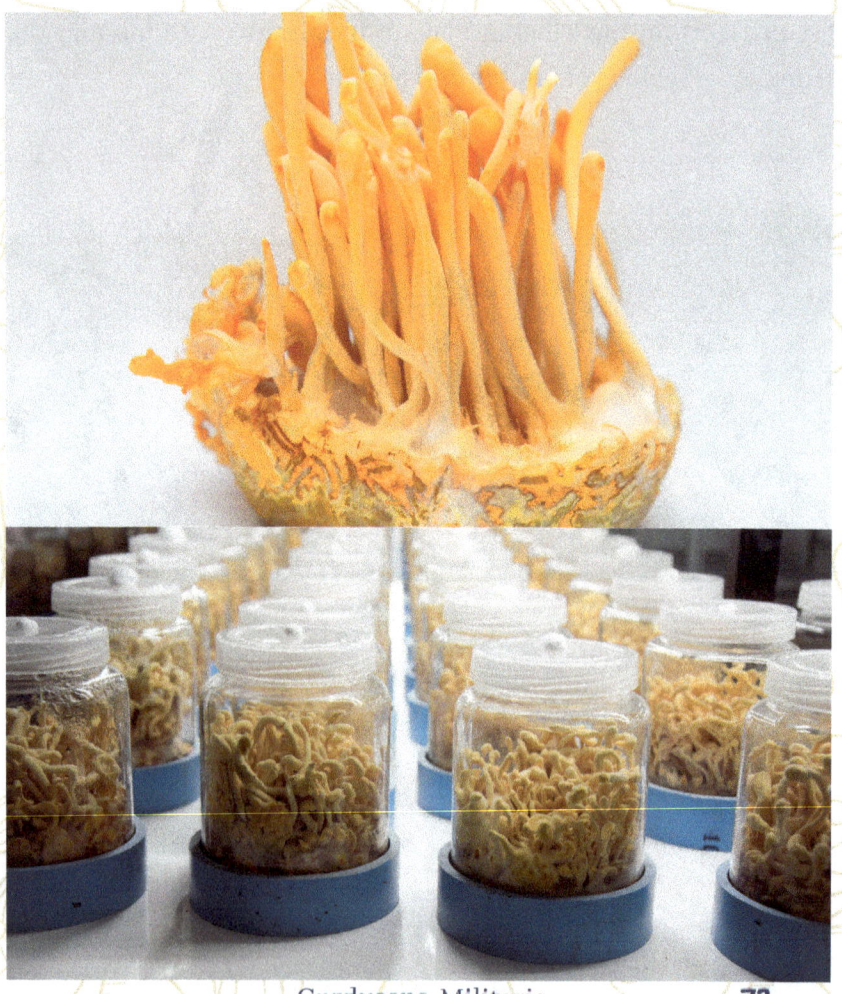

Cordyceps Militaris

6. Shiitake Mushroom

Shiitake mushrooms are found in Eastern Oriental countries such as Japan, normally growing on shii trees related to oaks. The mushrooms are currently expanded as well as harvested in America too.

Shiitake mushrooms are chocolaty brownish and black in color. They contrast with straw mushrooms, which are more grey or beige.

Shiitake mushrooms have a conventional mushroom form with an umbrella-shaped cap as well as a woody stem.

Shiitake mushrooms are harvested round the year.

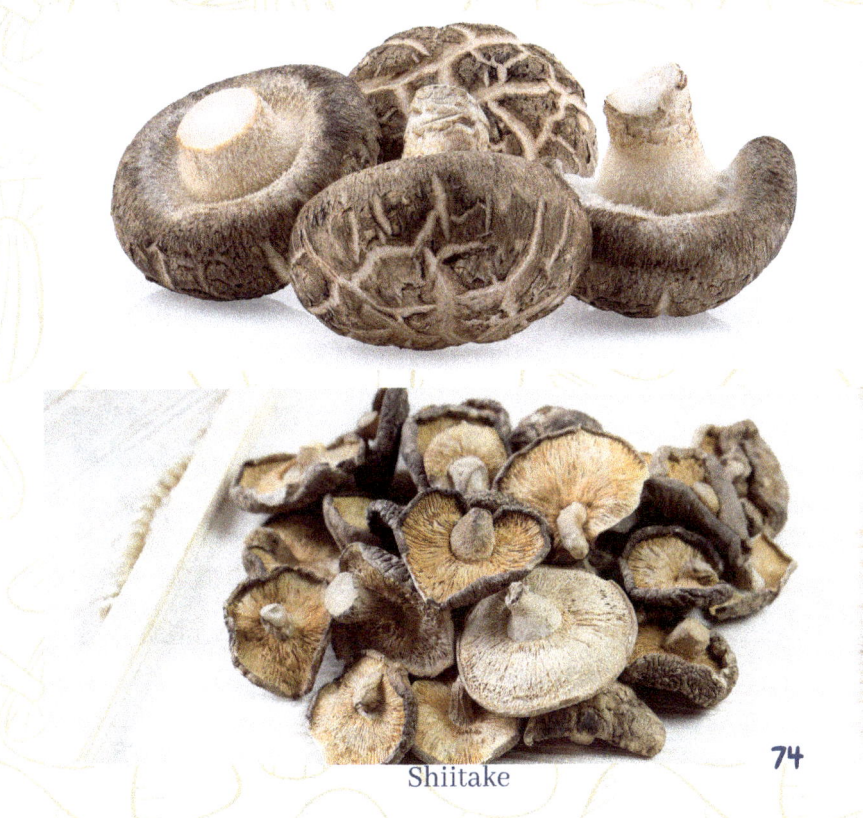

Shiitake

7. Maitake Mushroom : Hen of Woods

Maitake is a polypore bracket fungus that cultivates at the base of oak trees and other hardwoods in temperate forests from August to November. They are highly valued for both their medicinal effects and their cooking uses.

Maitake mushrooms grow in collections of squashed brown caps with white sides. The name "hen of the woods" originates from the cluster of mushrooms instead appears like the shaken up plumes of a sitting hen. Bigger maitake mushrooms transform a lighter tan, brownish or grey color as they develop. Each cap can be approximately 12" large, though sometimes you'll discover individual caps that are a lot larger than this. The top of the mushroom is commonly smooth and faintly wrinkled, and also, when fresh, its shade is bright orange to yellowish-orange.

With age, these mushroom caps will discolor and turn creamy colored, and become crumbly. Also, you can check that spot again in a couple of months or next year because this mushroom tends to fruit numerous times on the same log or tree. It is a polypore mushroom because its productive surface area (bottom) has various pores from where the spores are dispersed.

It suggests that there are no gills on the underside and that there will never be gills on the bottom. This mushroom always has a pore surface area with really tiny pores.

Maitake

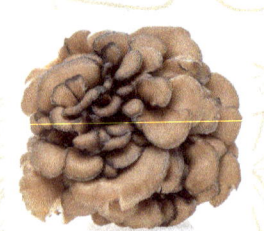

Photo by Maria Orlova from Pexels

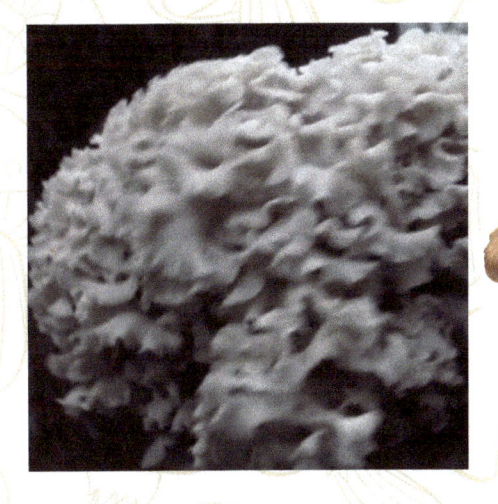

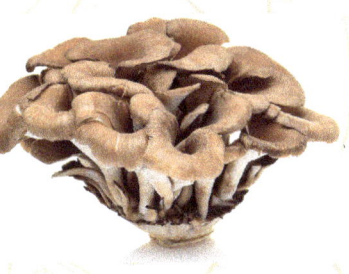

Cauliflower Mushroom (Lookalike)   Maitake

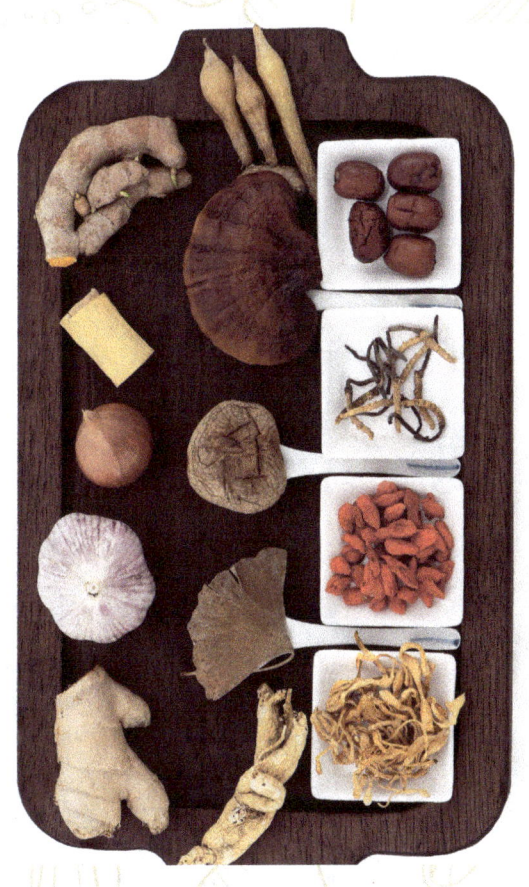

Medicinal Mushrooms

5. How to Take Medicinal Mushrooms

Advice is like mushrooms. The wrong kind can prove fatal.
- Charles E. McKenzie

Now that you know all the different benefits associated with medicinal mushrooms, you might be eager to get started. Using the information given in the earlier book of the series named "Mushroom Cultivation," you can grow the mushrooms you want at home itself. That said, these mushrooms can be sourced too. So let's look at the different options you can use for preparing and sourcing medicinal mushrooms.

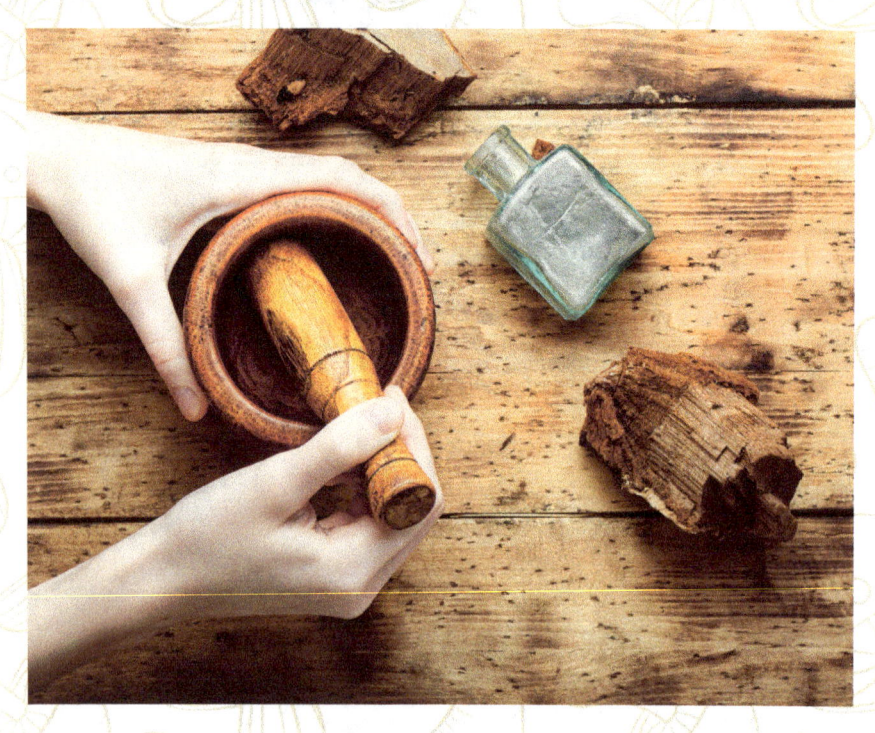

Making Chaga Powder

Preparing Medicinal Mushrooms

Medical mushrooms can be prepared in different ways. Depending on the mushrooms, you can either consume them fresh or in their dried forms.

Usually, the dried variants are preferred because the bioavailability of beneficial compounds in them is higher than their fresh counterparts. Also, the dosage varies depending on whether you are consuming fresh or dried mushrooms. You will need to consume more or fresh mushrooms than dried counterparts. Let's look at some different ways in which you can prepare medicinal mushrooms.

The most straightforward way to consume mushrooms is to cook them.

For instance, medicinal mushrooms such as button mushrooms, lion's mane, oyster mushrooms, enoki, maitake, and shiitake are ideal for cooking.

Depending on the flavor profile, you can add them to any recipe of your choice, such as a salad, soup, stew, or even stir-fry; these mushrooms come in handy.

Ensure that you don't cook them for a prolonged period. When you do this, they start losing their medicinal values. The ideal way to go about it is by simply flash-frying or roasting them.

If you are using dried mushrooms, they will need to be reconstituted for making elixirs or tinctures. This method is known as making a decoction.

This is also a simple way to consume polypore mushrooms. First, you need to heat water and place the mushrooms in them simply. You will need about a liter of water for two handfuls of mushrooms.

The hot water helps extract and break down the tough woody material of mushrooms, extract their medicinal compounds, and transform them into an absorbable form.

Brew the concoction you are making for at least 20-30 minutes. Then, whenever you want, you can always rebrew them. Feel free to store the brewed decoction in the fridge and use it whenever needed. You can also infuse the brew with helpful herbs of your choice, such as ginger.

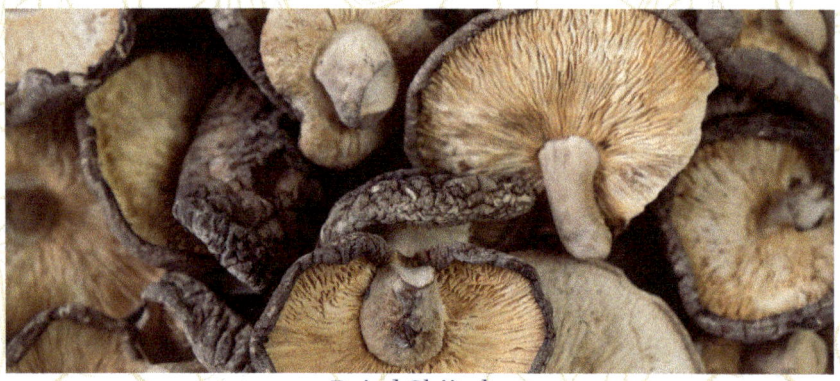

Dried Shiitake

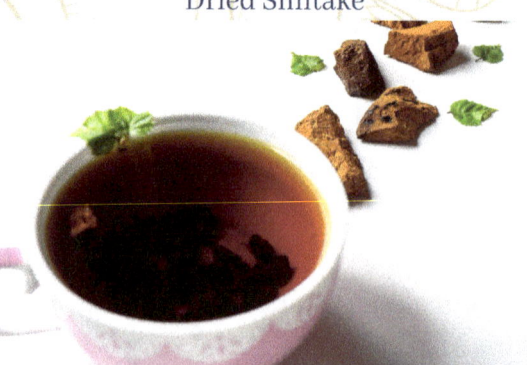

Chaga Tea

Dried mushrooms are also available in powdered form these days. If you are using mushroom powder, they will need to be added to different recipes of your choice. Certain mushrooms cannot be cooked with or found at local grocery stores such as reishi. Some medicinal ones taste quite unpleasant and cannot be consumed on their own. In such instances, opt for the powdered form. The powder can be used for making a tincture.

To increase the bioavailability of the medicinal constituent of mushrooms, the compounds are extracted using steam distillation and alcohol distillation. This ensures the active ingredients that are both soluble and insoluble in water are extracted from the mushrooms. Powdered mushrooms can be added to chocolates, salad dressings, or even used for baking.

Any alcohol tincture that's made with mushrooms makes the medicinal components in them more bioavailable for human consumption.

The good news is, making tinctures at home is quite easy. You need mushroom material of your choice, alcohol with at least 40% alcohol concentration, and some mason jars. Fill a jar with mushroom material so that it is 2/3 full. Then, fill the rest of it with alcohol.

Let this stand for two weeks while shaking it occasionally. After this, you need to strain the mushrooms out of the alcohol and bottom the map. These elixirs taste good on their own or can be combined with other recipes as well.

Sourcing Medicinal Mushrooms

You always have the option of growing medicinal mushrooms at home. If this option does not appeal to you for one reason or another, you can purchase mushroom supplements or high-quality mushroom formulas that are available on the market these days. However, when sourcing medicinal mushrooms, you need to be incredibly careful about the following.

The mushrooms, supplement, or product should be made only with the fruiting body and nothing else. It means the product shouldn't have any grains, stems, fillers, or mycelium. This is the best way to ensure you get most of the benefits offered by the specific mushroom. The fruiting body contains active phytochemicals, and it is the culmination of the entire fungal organism itself.

The concentration of beneficial active compounds, including polysaccharides such as beta-glucans, is highest in the fruiting body compared to the mycelium.

You should also pay attention to the level of beta-glucans present in the mushrooms. They are one of the most valuable active compounds, and check for this before purchasing any extract or a product.

If the mushroom extract or products are made with fruiting bodies, the levels of beta-glucan will naturally be high.

You should also pay attention to the extraction process used for deriving the beneficial compounds present in mushrooms; how the mushroom products are created matters a lot because this regulates the overall potency of the product.

Never purchase from any company that doesn't use scientific expertise for creating their supplements. Ideally, opt for mushroom products that are dual extracted. The first level of extraction is to obtain the beta-glucan present in the mushrooms. After this, the mushrooms go through another extraction process where ethanol brings out other constituents. When both these techniques are combined, it's known as dual extraction. When the mushrooms are dual extracted, the active compounds' bioavailability, absorbability, and even digestibility increase.

Apart from all this, you should always check the concentration of the number of capsules sold for finding your ideal dosage. Whenever you are purchasing a mushroom capsule, check how many capsules are there in it and the concentration of each capsule.

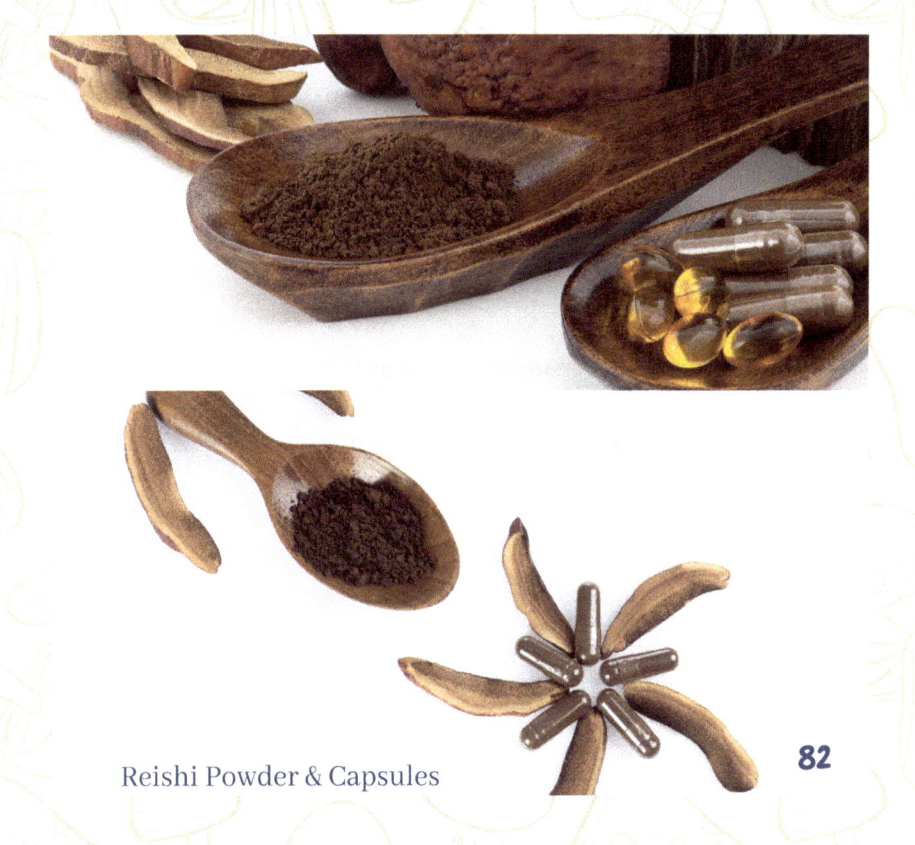

Reishi Powder & Capsules

While purchasing any mushroom supplements or products, ensure that you opt for a reliable and known supplier. The supplier should provide transparent and honest information about that extraction process and how they handle it. Any supplier who refuses to share this information with you is not reliable. When it comes to using medicinal mushrooms, the overall quality of the product matters; if there are any contaminants in it or the mushrooms are not handled properly, they can have adverse effects.

If you are foraging the mushrooms in the wild, ensure that you do it with an expert for this job. If not, you need to have all the required information to reduce the risk of accidentally consuming any inedible or poisonous variants. The problem is most mushrooms look quite similar. Some toxic variants look just like their helpful counterparts.

You can also visit a local farmer's market to purchase fresh or dried mushrooms.

Finally, don't forget to check the local health food stores for buying mushrooms.

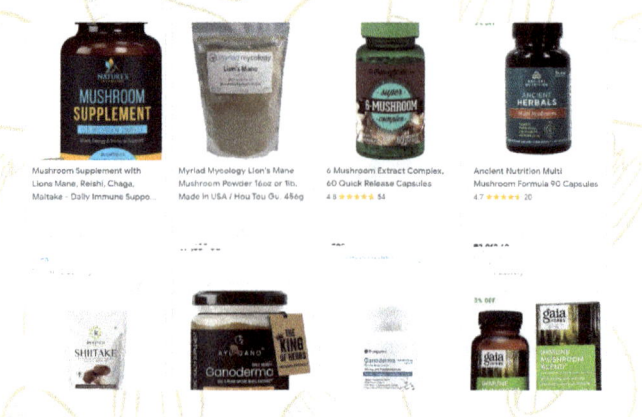

Mushroom supplements available online

6. How to cook Medicinal Mushrooms: 7 Recipes

The rich, hearty flavor of portobello mushroom caps is a dynamite alternative to the traditional burger
- Katie Lee

1. Chaga Tea

What you need :

- Clean Water
- Few Chaga pieces (4-5)
- Ginger, Cloves, Cinnamon, Cardamom (as per your taste and requirement)
- 1/3 tsp ground star anise
- 1/6 tsp black pepper
- 1/6 tsp stevia/sugar-free/honey or any sweetening agent as per your taste
- Some nut milk /cow milk

Steps:

- Start with a boiling pot with clean water on a sim flame and put Chaga pieces inside the pot.
- Depending on how strong you want to brew it, you can slowly heat it on a sim flame for a few more hours.
- Remember never to boil it.
- Add all other spices in the last 30 minutes of simmering.
- Once the brewing is complete, remove the Chaga chunk and store it in the freezer for 3-4 time reuse.

- Pore the brew in the bottle and store it in the refrigerator. You can use it for the next ten days.
- You can add stevia and a splash of milk (based on your choice) and serve it hot or cold.

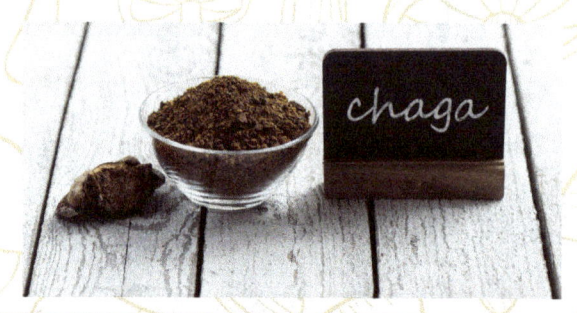

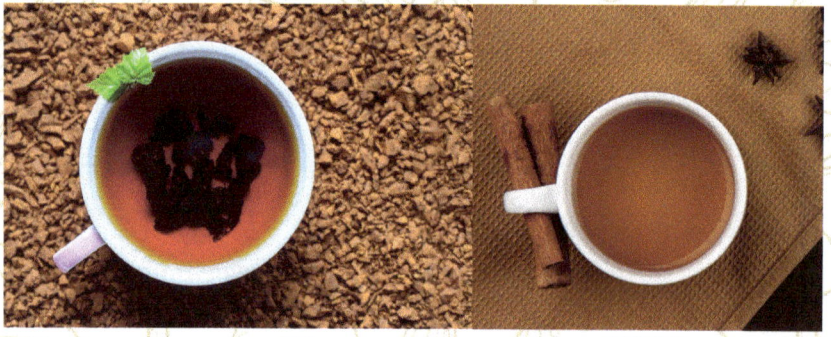

Chaga Tea without milk   Chaga Tea with milk splash

2. Golden Milk with Reishi

What you need :

- A tsp of Reishi Powder
- A cup of coconut milk (or any other milk you wish)
- 1 tsp Turmeric
- Ginger, Cloves, Cinnamon, Cardamom (as per your taste and requirement)
- 1/6 tsp black pepper
- 1/6 tsp stevia/sugar-free or any sweetening agent as per your taste.

Steps:

- In a pan, add milk, ginger, turmeric, and pepper. Apply sim flame while whisking periodically. Switch off heat, cover, and wait for 6-8 minutes.

- Use a blender to mix milk, reishi powder, and honey; blend until smooth and serve.

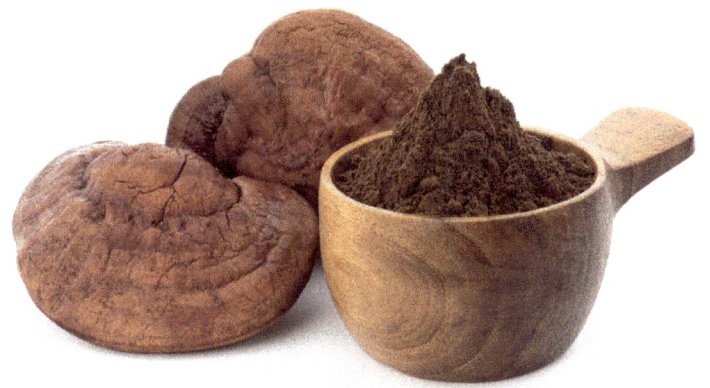

Reishi Powder

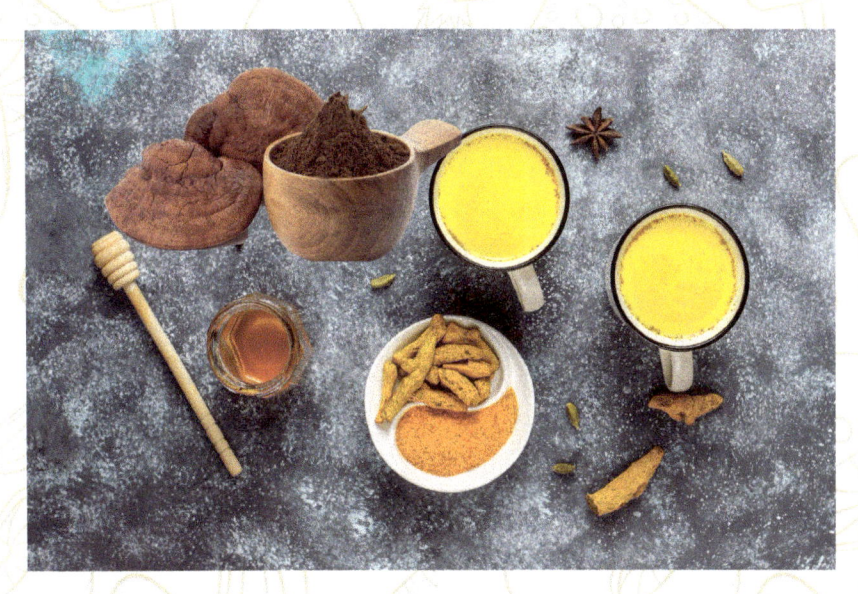

Golden Milk

3. Lion's Mane Nugget

What you need :

- 500 grams of lion's mane mushroom
- 1 cup chickpea flour
- 1 cup water
- 1 tsp garlic powder
- 1/2 tsp cumin
- 1/2 tsp coriander
- 1/2 tsp Indian Mix Spices (Garam Masala)

Steps :

- Pre-heat deep fryer to 180 degrees Celcius. Split up the lion's mane mushroom into bite-size.

- Extensively blend all dry ingredients. Flavors may be chosen relying on individual preference.

- Gradually add water until a damp batter is created. The batter will certainly thicken upon standing.

- Dip the pieces of lion's mane one by one permitting excess batter to drip right into the dish if adequately hot; the oil will bubble when the nugget is immersed.

- Fry for 8-10 mins till it becomes crisp and golden in color.

- Serve with mayonnaise or ketchup.

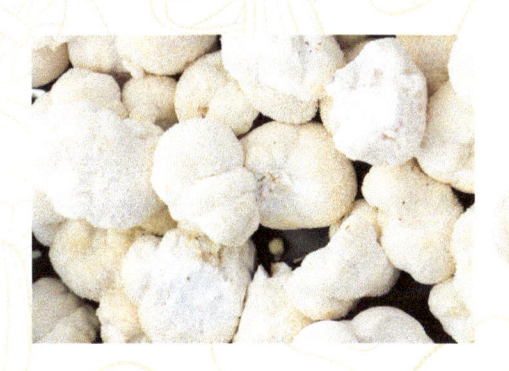

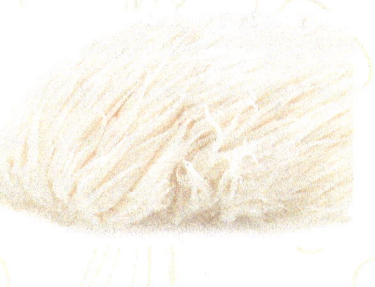

Bite Size Pieces

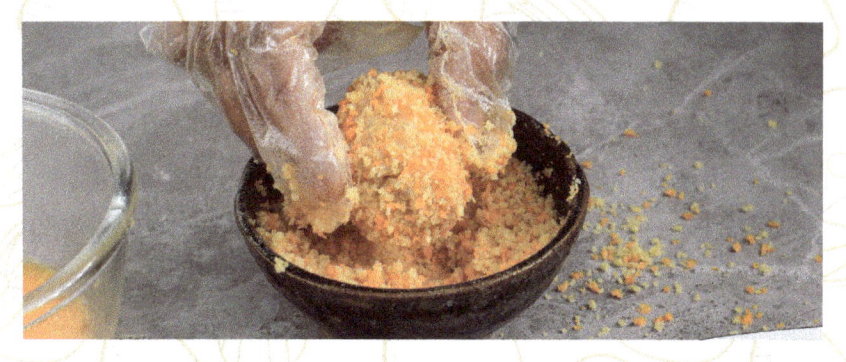

Dip in Batter

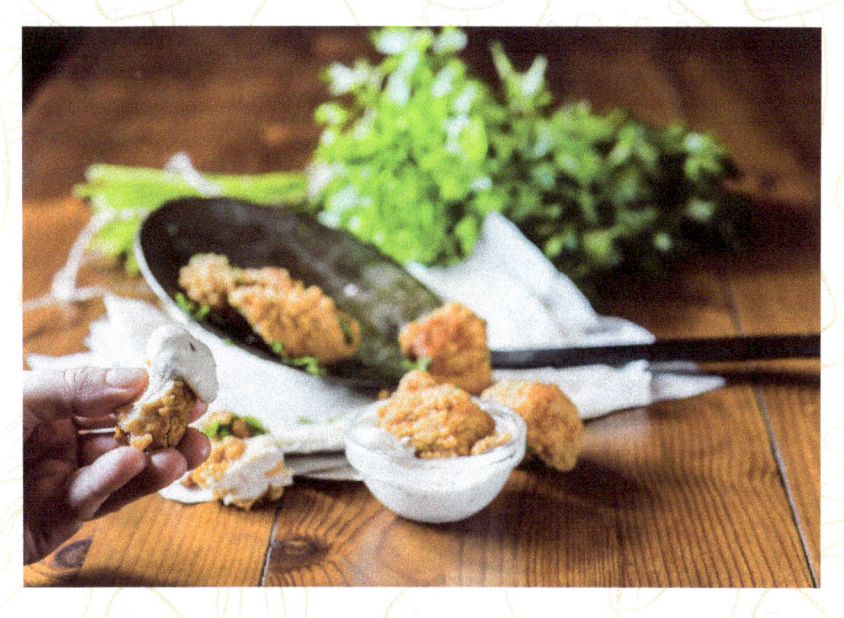

Serve Hot & Crispy

4. Turkey Tail Coffee

What you need :

- Around 400 gm of any Milk
- 4 ounces Fresh Brewed Strong Coffee or 2 Espresso shots
- 2 -3 tsp of Turkey Tail Powder
- 1-3 tsp of any Sweetener like Sugar, jaggery powder, Stevia, Honey, etc.

Steps :

- Pick up and make the coffee or espresso of your pick.
- While the coffee is preparing, heat the milk of your selection for 30-45 seconds in a microwave-safe coffee mug.
- Include Turkey tail powder and also stir it.
- When the milk is warmed, take a little whisk and vigorously whisk back and forth for 15-30 secs till the milk is foamy.

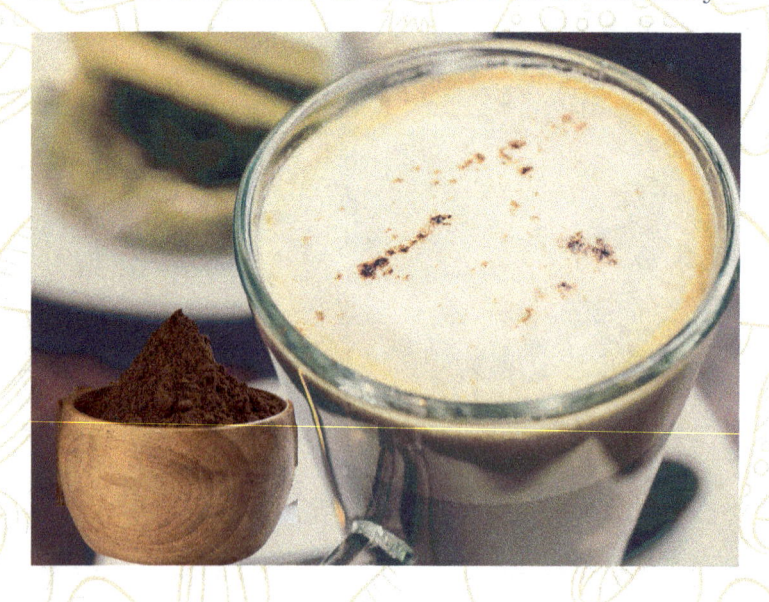

5. Cordyceps Biscuit

What you need :

- 2 eggs
- 1-3 tsp of any Sweetener like Sugar, jaggery powder, Stevia, Honey, etc.
- 1 cup almond flour
- 1/2 cup tapioca flour
- 1 teaspoon baking powder
- 2 -3 tsp of Cordyceps
- 1/2 Tbsp sea salt
- 1/2 cup cold ghee/butter
- 1 Tbsp apple cider vinegar
- 2 1/2 cups ultra-fine almond flour
- Ginger as per your taste
- 2 tsp cinnamon
- 1/2 tsp baking soda

Steps:

- Preheat stove to 400 levels Fahrenheit or 200 levels Celsius
- Line a baking sheet with parchment paper
- Blend all dry ingredients right into a mixing bowl and blend well. Gradually add honey and also ghee. Blend till all ingredients are mixed.
- Scoop a tablespoon sphere into your palm and place it on a baking sheet. Use your hand to flatten the mixture to your desired thickness gently. Repeat procedure.

- Bake for 10 mins or until cookies is a light golden brown around the sides.
- Take them out, and let the cookies cool down for 15 minutes.
- Offer as well as enjoy your delicious cookies!

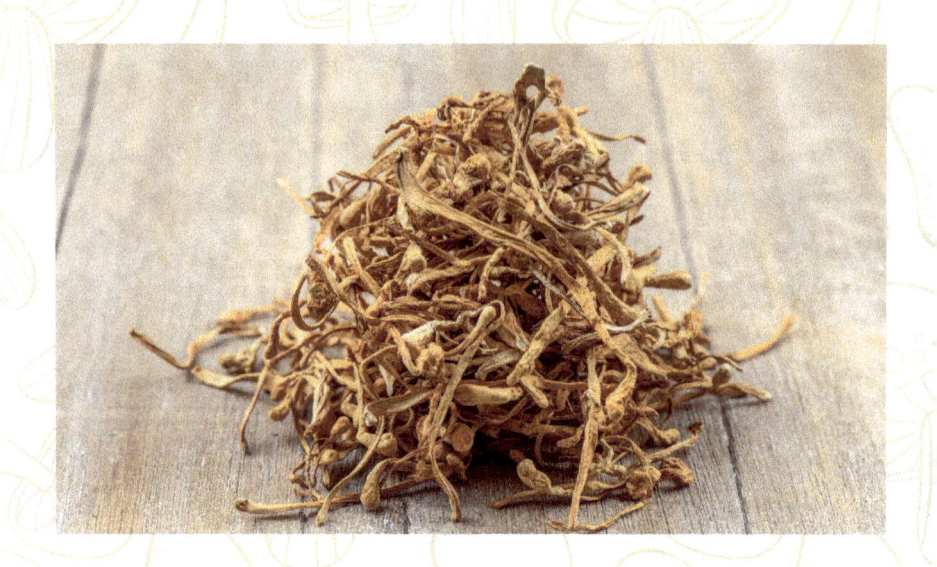

Dried Cordyceps

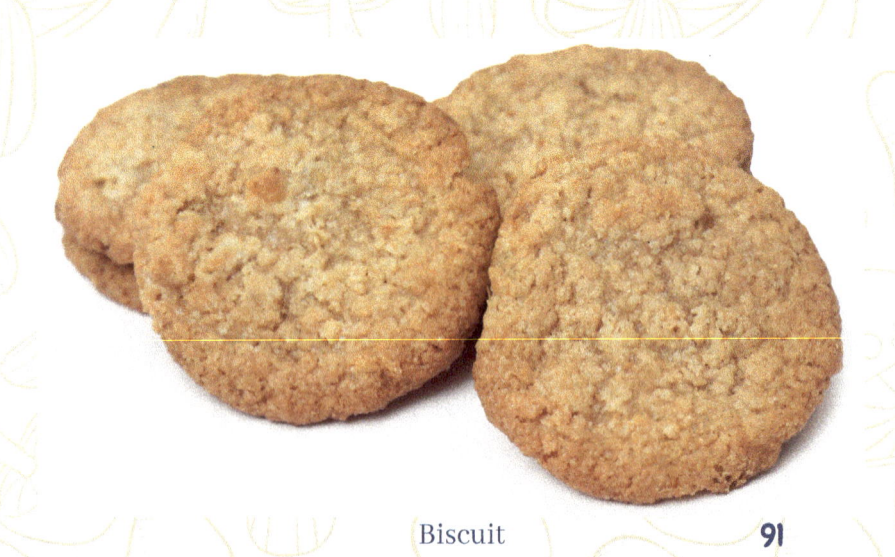

Biscuit

6. Baked Shiitake Side Dish

What you need :

- Shiitake Mushroom
- Garlic powder
- Salt
- Black Pepper
- Olive Oil
- White wine vinegar

Steps:

- Start with seasoning the mushrooms with a blend of olive oil, white wine vinegar, and spices of your choice.
- After that, you spread them on a rimmed baking sheet.
- Then bake them for about 20 mins in a 400 ° F oven.
- Garnish the dish with some parsley.
- Serve hot!

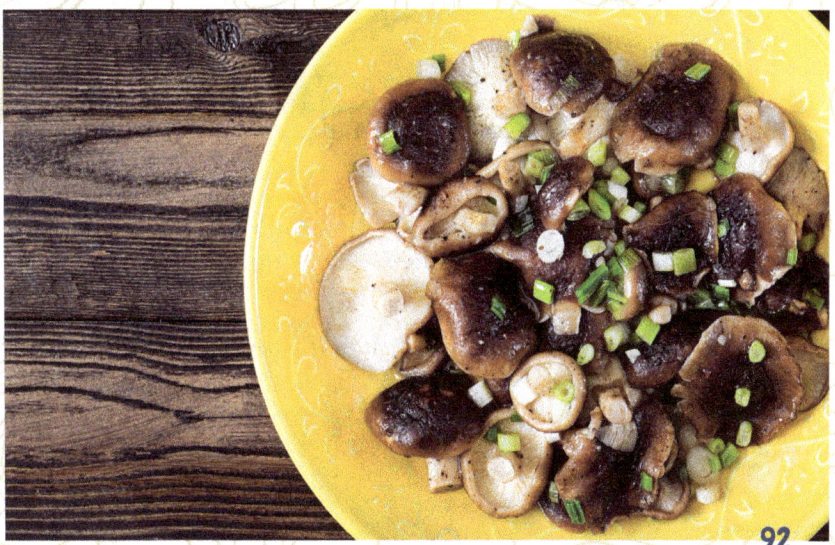

Shitake Side Dish

7. Maitake Pasta

What you need :

- Maitake mushroom
- Olive Oil
- White Wine
- Sour cream/crème fraîche

Steps:

- Keep a large pot of water to a boil over medium-high flame. Add the pasta and boil for 8 minutes. Drain the pasta.

- Heat a pan over medium heat, add two tablespoons of olive oil, and heat through. Add the mushrooms and sauté until they turn golden brown in about 3-4 minutes.

- Return the pan to medium heat, add the remaining olive oil, and put the garlic and shallots in it, occasionally stirring, till the shallots are tender.

- Add the wine and let it reduce to half.

- Blend in the crème fraîche until integrated, mix in the Parmesan & after that, season with salt and pepper.

- Add the sauce of choice and garnish it with cheese.

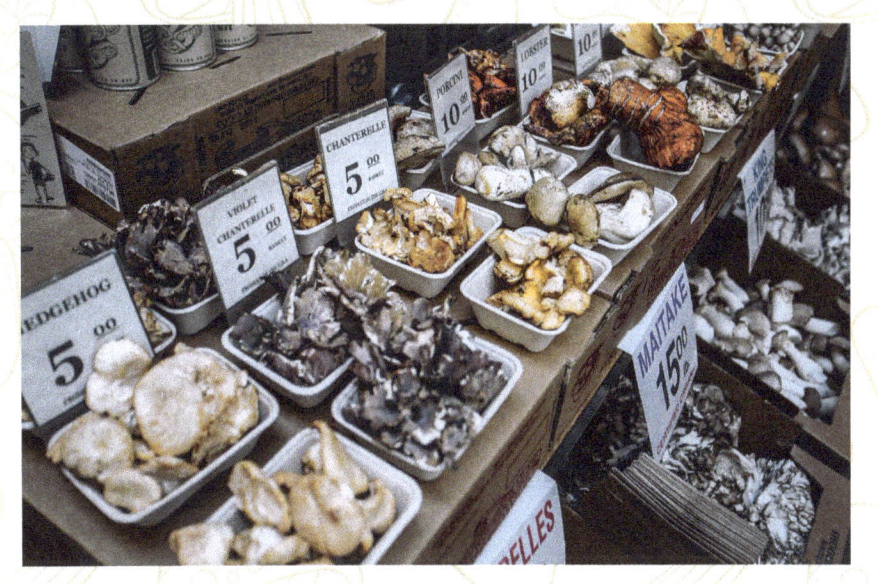

Maitake Mushroom in a Local Store

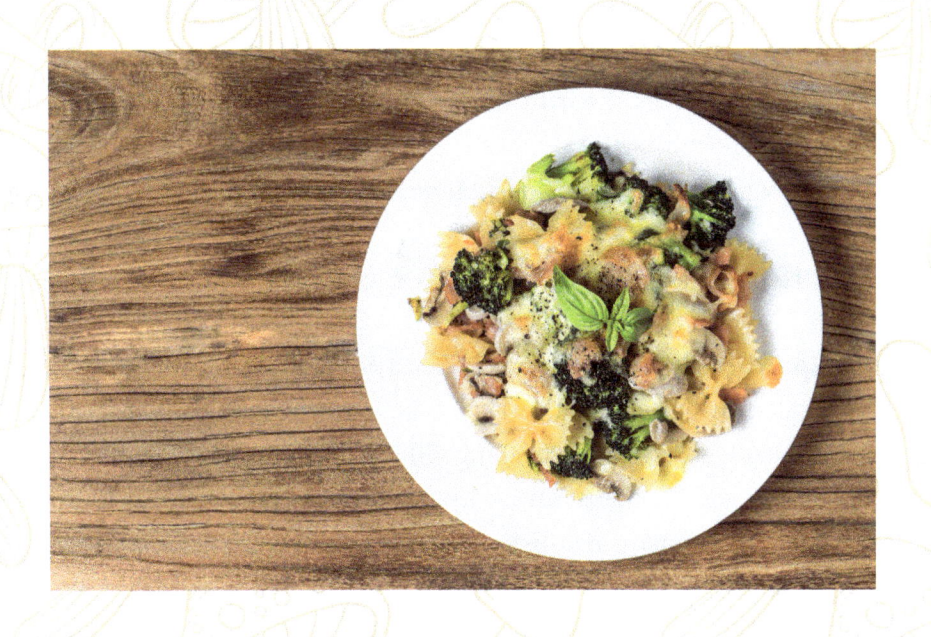

Maitake Pasta

7. Frequently Asked Questions (FAQ) & Glossary

You have to treat yourself like a mushroom to some degree, in order to keep on discovering things.

— Christian Bale

Q1.

I found a 12 pound Lion's Mane recently and saved half of it for dehydrating. I just finished processing it all into powder.

I initially planned to make capsules but stored them in air-tight jars due to the possibility of moisture getting in. Also, the tincture process seems quite complex.

Then I read that the mycelium holds most of the nootropic compounds and not the fruiting body.

So, what should I do with Lion's Mane powder?

Solutions

- You can likewise sterilize it for a longer life span. Leave it sealed in the jar, dual turkey bag, and put it in the pressure cooker at 15 psi for an hr. You will break down the chitin, make it very easy to digest and keep the nutritional worths and the long-chain medical substances-- an extra 'entire food' strategy to supplementation.

- You can make a tincture by submerging it in 60% alcohol with 1 part mushroom to 3 parts alcohol for fresh mushroom, or one part dried mushroom to 5 parts 40% alcohol for dried mushroom.

- There are lots of YouTube videos regarding dual extractions if you wish to learn. I have a lion's mane tincture macerating now. Alcohol extraction initially for 3 months, and then simmer very same product in water for a couple of hrs. Strain as well as incorporate them for a double extraction. It's pretty direct.

- Tincturing is very simple. Dry it, grind it right into a powder, let it sit in alcohol for 2-3 months. Different the grounds, then position them in hot water for 8-10hrs. Combine alcohol as well as hot water.

- You can make pills,25 grams each, then vacuum cleaner seal them, and also put them in containers in the freezer until usage. I do batches of 100 as that's what my tablet manufacturer does, so I only have 100 out each time.

Q2.

Concern regarding Chaga tincture.

I plan to make a double extraction(DE). Up until I had time to research the correct technique for making the DE, I had actually been making tea with it. I have actually recycled this batch of Chaga for a few batches of tea. Because I've currently used up the water-soluble components, I would love to make a tincture. What is the very best approach?

Solutions

Do a triple extract. First, macerate mushrooms in 190 proof ethanol for 24 hours.

Next, strain and set ethanol aside. Put the mushrooms in a crockpot with distilled water on low for two days. 1/2 the water will evaporate.

Next, pour mushrooms and water back into the ethanol mixture and let sit for two weeks.

If you put 1/2 the amount of water that you have for alcohol, it will be 40% alcohol. You don't want more water than alcohol.

You can buy organic 190 proof cane ethanol in bulk. I make my tinctures in large mason jars and then bottle them.

Q3.
I live in the UK, and I'm struggling to find Cordyceps and Lion's Mane tinctures?

Solutions
Few options where you can check and decide. (Note: I have no relationship with the below companies, it was suggested by some UK users).

- https://www.biovea.com/uk
- vitalherbs.co.uk

Q4.
What is Mushroom Tincture and Double Extraction?

Solutions

An extract is made by soaking the mushroom in any solvents, such as vinegar, water, or alcohol. This process draws out the active components to have a better result on your body.

A tincture is when we primarily use alcohol to soak the mushroom. The word tincture and also extract are used as same. Yet they're not the same thing. The distinction is majorly on the manufacturing process.

Double Extraction means the mushroom is soaked in alcohol and then in hot water, which extracts different qualities from the mushroom. Some individuals utilize a triple extraction which indicates an initial cold-water soak is performed.

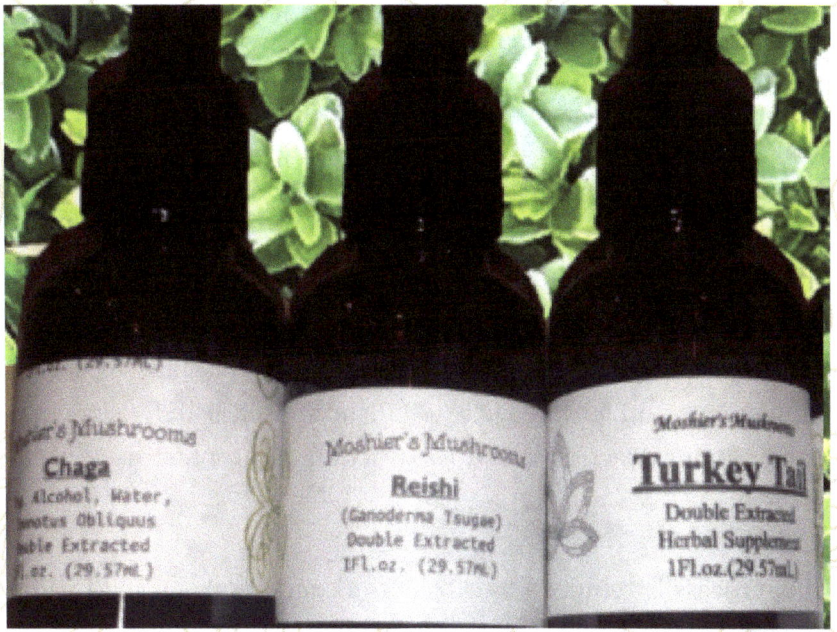

Mushroom Tinctures

Glossary

Active Compounds
Active compounds are found in food with an organic effect or wellness advantage for the person consuming it.

Adaptogens
Adaptogens are commonly occurring non-toxic materials that make our bodies durable to stress factors, whether physical, mental, ecological, or chemical, by harmonizing and optimizing our physical functions. The prime systems they regulate are the endocrine, nerve system, immune, digestion, and cardio functions.

Substrate
You can consider substrate as the "dirt" the mushrooms grow in.

For gourmet or medical mushrooms, the substrate is usually wood, with some kind of nutritional booster like wheat bran or oat bran. Occasionally mushrooms are grown on logs, in which case the substrate is just the log itself.

Some mushrooms, like the typical switch mushroom, are "main decomposers", indicating they will be expanded on a substrate of compost.

Extraction
The extraction method is used in any sort of plant or fungi supplement, and with regards to mushrooms, it usually refers to warm water extraction, alcohol extraction, or in some cases, both of them.

This process is required to extract the compounds locked inside mushrooms. (Alcohol, water, or both may be used)

For example, Beta-glucans are soluble in water, but other compounds are soluble in alcohol.

Fruiting Body

It is the part of the mushroom that outgrows the ground, tree or log, and is likewise the part of the mushroom that can generate spores. So, if you have ever seen a mushroom at the grocery store, you are taking a look at the fruiting body!

The fruiting body consists of high quantities of valuable beta-glucans as well as other critical bioactive substances.

Mycelium

The mycelium is the underground part of a fungus. It is made up of hyphae, which look like strings or rootlets. The floor covering of hyphae might be extremely heavily woven. Its major function is to draw out nutrients.

Cap

Top of the fruiting body that is seen over the ground as well as where the spores originate from.

Agar in Mushrooming

Agar is utilized in the cultivation of mushrooms in order to save cultures for long-lasting use and save them from being contaminated. Spores are germinated on agar before clean transfer to the new agar plate.

Spores

Spores are like the "seeds" of the mushroom.

The spore contains half of the genetic material required for the mushroom mycelium to form and the mushroom to grow ultimately.

Spores are available in various sizes and shapes and are sometimes a robust method to identify different types of mushrooms through Spore Printing.

Spore Print

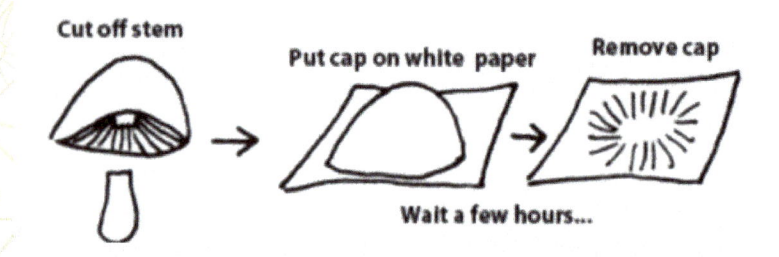

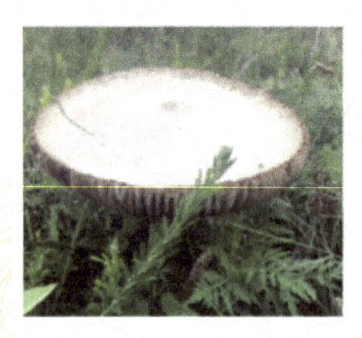

Cut off stem → **Put cap on white paper** → **Remove cap**

Wait a few hours...

The Mushroom

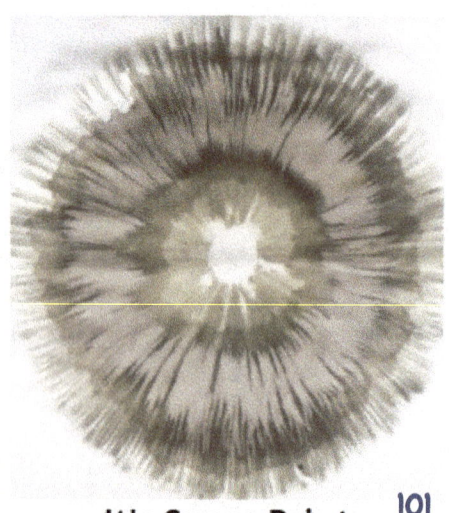

It's Spore Print

8. Conclusion

I want to thank you once again for choosing this book. I hope it proved to be an enjoyable and informative read.

In this book, you were introduced to various medicinal mushrooms and the different health benefits they offer.

The growing scientific body of research into understanding mushrooms' healing and medicinal properties is finally helping us understand that true potential.

From reducing the severity of allergic symptoms and increasing antioxidants in the body to regulating inflammation, improving cardiovascular health, and supporting immune function, medicinal mushrooms offer different benefits.

This book will act as your guide to understand all the health benefits you can gain by using different types of mushrooms.

Apart from this, you were also introduced to simple tips and suggestions that will come in handy for identifying and sourcing medicinal mushrooms. Also, seven recipes have been provided for cooking the medicinal mushroom of your choice.

Thank you and all the best!

9. References

5 Top Mushroom Growing Supplies You Need for Your Mushroom Farm. (n.d.). Fungi Ally. Https://www.fungially.com/blogs/growing-mushrooms/5-top-mushroom-growing-supplies-need-mushroom-farm

9 Tips For Your First Mushroom Trip. (n.d.). Www.24high.com. https://www.24high.com/en/blog/14/9-TIPS-FOR-A-BEGINNER-FIRST-MAGIC-MUSHROOMS-TRIP

Abdel-Monem, N. M., El-Saadani, M. A., Daba, A. S., Saleh, S. R., & Aleem, E. (2020). Exopolysaccharide-peptide complex from oyster mushroom (Pleurotus ostreatus) protects against hepatotoxicity in rats. Biochemistry and Biophysics Reports, 24, 100852. https://doi.org/10.1016/j.bbrep.2020.100852

Amsterdam, J. van, Opperhuizen, A., & Brink, W. van den. (2011). Harm potential of magic mushroom use: A review. Regulatory Toxicology and Pharmacology, 59(3), 423–429. https://doi.org/10.1016/j.yrtph.2011.01.006

Choi, S. Y., Hur, S. J., An, C. S., Jeon, Y. H., Jeoung, Y. J., Bak, J. P., & Lim, B. O. (2010, March 10). Anti-Inflammatory Effects of Inonotus obliquus in Colitis Induced by Dextran Sodium Sulfate. Journal of Biomedicine and Biotechnology. https://www.hindawi.com/journals/bmri/2010/943516/

Chu, T. T. W., Benzie, I. F. F., Lam, C. W. K., Fok, B. S. P., Lee, K. K. C., & Tomlinson, B. (2012). Study of potential cardioprotective effects of Ganoderma lucidum (Lingzhi): results of a controlled human intervention trial. The British Journal of Nutrition, 107(7), 1017–1027. https://doi.org/10.1017/S0007114511003795

Cohut, M. (2019, March 15). Does eating mushrooms protect brain health? Www.medicalnewstoday.com. https://www.medicalnewstoday.com/articles/324710#A-dramatic-effect-on-cognitive-decline?

Cui, X.-Y., Cui, S.-Y., Zhang, J., Wang, Z.-J., Yu, B., Sheng, Z.-F., Zhang, X.-Q., & Zhang, Y.-H. (2012). Extract of Ganoderma lucidum prolongs sleep time in rats. Journal of Ethnopharmacology, 139(3), 796–800. https://doi.org/10.1016/j.jep.2011.12.020

Dicks, L., & Ellinger, S. (2020). Effect of the Intake of Oyster Mushrooms (Pleurotus ostreatus) on Cardiometabolic Parameters—A Systematic Review of Clinical Trials. Nutrients, 12(4). https://doi.org/10.3390/nu12041134

Feng, L., Cheah, I. K.-M., Ng, M. M.-X., Li, J., Chan, S. M., Lim, S. L., Mahendran, R., Kua, E.-H., & Halliwell, B. (2019). The Association between Mushroom Consumption and Mild Cognitive Impairment: A Community-Based Cross-Sectional Study in Singapore. Journal of Alzheimer's Disease, 68(1), 197–203. https://doi.org/10.3233/jad-180959

Freeman, S., & Chandler, N. (2009, February 25). How Magic Mushrooms Work. HowStuffWorks. https://science.howstuffworks.com/magic-mushroom6.htm

Ganesan, K., & Xu, B. (2019). Anti-Diabetic Effects and Mechanisms of Dietary Polysaccharides. Molecules (Basel, Switzerland), 24(14), 2556. https://doi.org/10.3390/molecules24142556

Garza, E. (2020, May 31). How to Naturally Relieve Allergies. Om Mushroom Superfood. https://ommushrooms.com/blogs/blog/how-to-naturally-relieve-allergies

Growing Mushrooms Indoors - A Full Guide | Gardening Tips. (n.d.). Gardeningtips.in. Https://gardeningtips.in/growing-mushrooms-indoors-a-full-guide

Heart Health. (n.d.). Mushrooms Canada. https://www.mushrooms.ca/health-concerns/mushrooms-and-heart-health/

How Many Different Types of Psychedelic Mushrooms Are There? (2019, June 15). Psychedelic Invest. https://psychedelicinvest.com/how-many-different-types-of-psychedelic-mushrooms-are-there/

How do Mushrooms Support the Immune System? (2020, May 28). Real Mushrooms. https://www.realmushrooms.com/mushrooms-immune-system/

Jayachandran, M., Xiao, M., & Xu, J. (2017). Health Promoting Benefits of Edible Mushrooms through Gut Microbiota. Www.sciepub.com. http://www.sciepub.com/reference/255169

Jeong, S. C., Jeong, Y. T., Yang, B. Y., Islam, R., Koyyalamudi, S., Pang, G., Cho, K. Y., & Song, C. H. (2010). White button mushroom (Agaricus bisporus) lowers blood glucose and cholesterol levels in diabetic and hypercholesterolemic rats. Nutrition Research, 30(1), 49–56. https://doi.org/10.1016/j.nutres.2009.12.003

Kabir, Y., & Kimura, S. (1989). Dietary mushrooms reduce blood pressure in spontaneously hypertensive rats(SHR). Journal of Nutritional Science and Vitaminology, 35(1), 91–94. https://doi.org/10.3177/jnsv.35.91

Different Types of Mushrooms and Their Uses. (n.d.). Www.mushroom-Appreciation.com. Https://www.mushroom-appreciation.com/types-of-mushrooms.html#sthash.8duqpi6r.dpbs

The Journal of Clinical Endocrinology & Metabolism, 104(10), 4837–4847. https://doi.org/10.1210/jc.2018-01791

Richman, E. L., Kenfield, S. A., Stampfer, M. J., Giovannucci, E. L., Zeisel, S. H., Willett, W. C., & Chan, J. M. (2012). Choline intake and risk of lethal prostate cancer: incidence and survival. The American Journal of Clinical Nutrition, 96(4), 855–863. https://doi.org/10.3945/ajcn.112.039784

Sessa, B., & Johnson, M. W. (2015). Can psychedelic compounds play a part in drug dependence therapy?. The British journal of psychiatry : the journal of mental science, 206(1), 1–3. https://doi.org/10.1192/bjp.bp.114.148031

Schneider, I., Kressel, G., Meyer, A., Krings, U., Berger, R. G., & Hahn, A. (2011). Lipid lowering effects of oyster mushroom (Pleurotus ostreatus) in humans. Journal of Functional Foods, 3(1), 17–24. https://doi.org/10.1016/j.jff.2010.11.004

Sima, P., Vannucci, L., & Vetvicka, V. (2018). β-glucans and cholesterol (Review). International Journal of Molecular Medicine. https://doi.org/10.3892/ijmm.2018.3411

Schneider, I., Kressel, G., Meyer, A., Krings, U., Berger, R. G., & Hahn, A. (2011). Lipid lowering effects of oyster mushroom (Pleurotus ostreatus) in humans. Journal of Functional Foods, 3(1), 17–24. https://doi.org/10.1016/j.jff.2010.11.004
Six Steps to Mushroom Farming. (n.d.). Mushroom Council. https://www.mushroomcouncil.com/growing-mushrooms/six-steps-to-mushroom-farming/

Sun, S., Li, X., Ren, A., Du, M., Du, H., Shu, Y., Zhu, L., & Wang, W. (2016). Choline and betaine consumption lowers cancer risk: a meta-analysis of epidemiologic studies. Scientific Reports, 6(1). https://doi.org/10.1038/srep35547

Tanaka, A., Nishimura, M., Sato, Y., Sato, H., & Nishihira, J. (2016). Enhancement of the Th1-phenotype immune system by the intake of Oyster mushroom (Tamogitake) extract in a double-blind, placebo-controlled study. Journal of Traditional and Complementary Medicine, 6(4), 424–430. https://doi.org/10.1016/j.jtcme.2015.11.004

The Benefits of Chaga Mushroom. (n.d.). Super U. https://superu.co.uk/blogs/news/chaga-mushroom-health-benefits

Urbancikova, I., Hudackova, D., Majtan, J., Rennerova, Z., Banovcin, P., & Jesenak, M. (2020). Efficacy of Pleuran (β-Glucan from Pleurotus ostreatus) in the Management of Herpes Simplex Virus Type 1 Infection. Evidence-Based Complementary and Alternative Medicine, 2020, 1–8. https://doi.org/10.1155/2020/8562309

Kalaras, M. D., Richie, J. P., Calcagnotto, A., & Beelman, R. B. (2017). Mushrooms: A rich source of the antioxidants ergothioneine and glutathione. Food Chemistry, 233, 429–433. https://doi.org/10.1016/j.foodchem.2017.04.109

Lang, A. (2020, January 6). Are Mushrooms Good for Diabetes? Healthline. https://www.healthline.com/nutrition/mushrooms-good-for-diabetes#benefits

Leslie, M. G. (2018, August 7). 11 of the Best Mushroom Kits to Grow Your Own | Gardener's Path. Gardener's Path. Https://gardenerspath.com/plants/vegetables/best-mushroom-growing-kits/

Maldonado, E. (2019, March 10). The Mushroom Life Cycle. Forest Origins. https://forestorigins.com/blogs/mushroom-blog-posts/the-mushroom-life-cycle

McRae, M. P. (2018). Dietary Fiber Intake and Type 2 Diabetes Mellitus: An Umbrella Review of Meta-analyses. Journal of Chiropractic Medicine, 17(1), 44–53. https://doi.org/10.1016/j.jcm.2017.11.002

Mel. (2018, October 29). My Mushroom Growing Supplies List. Mel's Garden. Https://wheelbarrowexpert.com/my-mushroom-growing-supplies-list/

Mulcahy, L. (2019, June 3). 6 Health Benefits of Mushrooms That Will Surprise You. Good Housekeeping. https://www.goodhousekeeping.com/health/diet-nutrition/a27633487/mushroom-health-benefits/

Mushrooms 4 Mental Health - Mushrooms 4 Life Blog. (2020, May 19). https://mushrooms4life.com/mushrooms-4-mental-health/

Nagano, M., Shimizu, K., Kondo, R., Hayashi, C., Sato, D., Kitagawa, K., & Ohnuki, K. (2010). Reduction of depression and anxiety by 4 weeks Hericium erinaceus intake. Biomedical Research (Tokyo, Japan), 31(4), 231–237. https://doi.org/10.2220/biomedres.31.231

Parker, B. (2020, September 6). Mushroom Structure: What are the Basic Parts of a Mushroom? Mushroom Site. https://mushroomsite.com/2020/09/06/parts-of-a-mushroom/

Plows, J., Stanley, J., Baker, P., Reynolds, C., & Vickers, M. (2018). The Pathophysiology of Gestational Diabetes Mellitus. International Journal of Molecular Sciences, 19(11), 3342. https://doi.org/10.3390/ijms19113342

Poddar, K. H., Ames, M., Hsin-Jen, C., Feeney, M. J., Wang, Y., & Cheskin, L. J. (2013). Positive effect of mushrooms substituted for meat on body weight, body composition, and health parameters. A 1-year randomized clinical trial. Appetite, 71, 379–387. https://doi.org/10.1016/j.appet.2013.09.008

Porter, K. M., Ward, M., Hughes, C. F., O'Kane, M., Hoey, L., McCann, A., Molloy, A. M., Cunningham, C., Casey, M. C., Tracey, F., Strain, S., McCarroll, K., Laird, E., Gallagher, A. M., & McNulty, H. (2019). Hyperglycemia and Metformin Use Are Associated With B Vitamin Deficiency and Cognitive Dysfunction in Older Adults.

Yao, W., Zhang, J., Dong, C., Zhuang, C., Hirota, S., Inanaga, K., & Hashimoto, K. (2015). Effects of amycenone on serum levels of tumor necrosis factor-α, interleukin-10, and depression-like behavior in mice after lipopolysaccharide administration. Pharmacology Biochemistry and Behavior, 136, 7–12. https://doi.org/10.1016/j.pbb.2015.06.012

Yang, S., Yan, Yang, L., Meng, Y., Wang, N., He, C., Fan, Y., & Zhou, Y. (2019, April 1). Alkali-soluble Polysaccharides From Mushroom Fruiting Bodies Improve Insulin Resistance. International Journal of Biological Macromolecules. https://pubmed.ncbi.nlm.nih.gov/30594618/

Young, M. R. I., & Xiong, Y. (2018). Influence of vitamin D on cancer risk and treatment: Why the variability? Trends in Cancer Research, 13, 43–53. https://www.ncbi.nlm.nih.gov/pmc/articles/PMC6201256/

Yu, S., Wu, X., Ferguson, M., Simmen, R. C., Cleves, M. A., Simmen, F. A., & Fang, N. (2016). Diets Containing Shiitake Mushroom Reduce Serum Lipids and Serum Lipophilic Antioxidant Capacity in Rats123. The Journal of Nutrition, 146(12), 2491–2496. https://doi.org/10.3945/jn.116.239806

DIY MUSHROOM SERIES

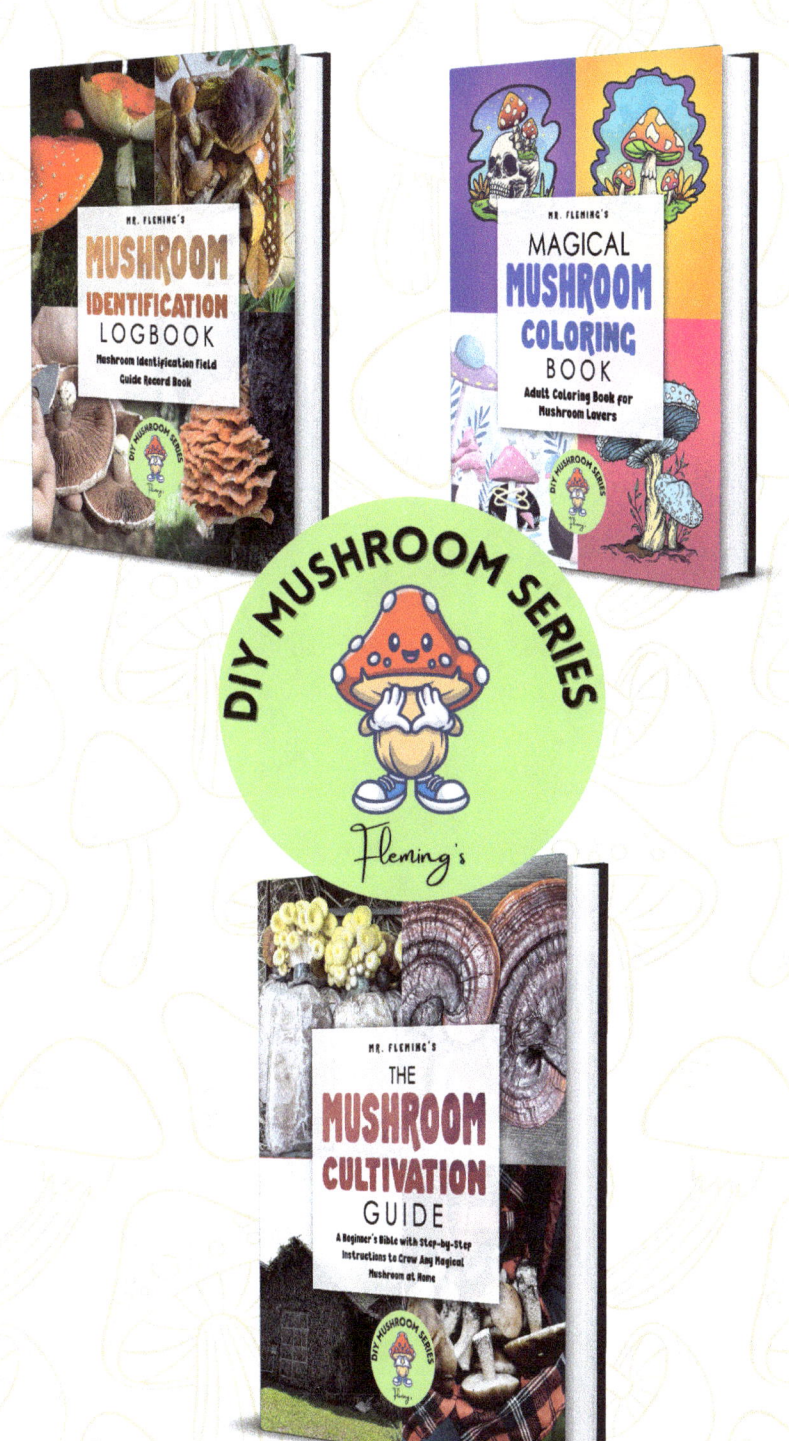

Mr. Fleming's Mushroom Identification Logbook
Mushroom Identification Field Guide Record Book

Mr. Fleming's Magical Mushroom Coloring Book
Adult Coloring Book for Mushroom Lovers

Mr. Fleming's The Mushroom Cultivation Guide
A Beginner's Bible with Step-by-Step Instructions to Grow Any Magical Mushroom at Home

Fleming's